SURVIVING YOUR OWN HOLOCAUST

SURVIVING YOUR OWN HOLOCAUST

From Litchfield versus a College
of SOME Physicians and Surgeons

Dr. Bryant F. Litchfield, MD

Library of Congress Control Number:		2010916607
ISBN:	Hardcover	978-1-4568-1206-5
	Softcover	978-1-4568-1205-8
	Ebook	978-1-4568-1207-2

This book was printed in the United States of America.

To order additional copies of this book, contact:
Xlibris Corporation
1-888-795-4274
www.Xlibris.com
Orders@Xlibris.com
84660

Contents

This book is dedicated to my wife, Dianne, who died in November 2008, and to my children Becky, Michael, Amy, Leisl, Shawn, David, Cameron, Marcus, and Keltie who have determined to continue to be a close extended family and to love, laugh with, and help each other – choosing to fill in some of the gaps left by their mother's departure – so that their family can go on.

PREFACE

Power is revealed not in striking hard or often,
but in striking true.
– Honoré De Balzac

It has been suggested that I gather up knowledge of all the facts,
and sufferings and abuses put upon me and my family . . .
and also the names of all persons that have had a hand in our
oppressions, as far as I can get hold of them and find them out.
– Personal source

HELLO, MY NAME is Bryant. I was a licensed physician in a province in Canada from 1986 to 2008. Then my license to practice was taken from me. The process by which my license was taken was my most recent personal holocaust. I started to write "final holocaust," but then I realized that I may still face some more challenges in life. I have decided to write a book about getting through these life challenges. Actually, this IS the book. Its purposes are as follows:

- To tell my family's story. From 1989, the media published their torrid version of my story. Their purpose was never to expose the truth, but to sell their product usually by printing *whatever had been said by someone*. They had almost no information from me but tried to tell my story. It really didn't work. In 2008, the college in my province published their incriminating summary of the most recent chapter of my story in the college newsletter. As you will see, their version was so confounded by unjust procedural techniques that they got no closer to the truth than the sensationalist media. I think, now, it's my turn to tell *my story*. I suspect it will be a tad different from those other two versions.

- To teach the difference between crying and weeping: both involve tears and grief. However, when you cry, your eyes close and you shut the world out. When you weep, your eyes are open – you share your grief with the world. I have learned to weep, and I will do this in sharing my story with you.

- To tell about the survival of my family and myself through inordinate trials, even as we lost my dear wife at only fifty-three.

- To review methods of breast exam so that readers, medical and nonmedical, can talk freely about "best practice" and variations in practice. The appalling truth is that one local "expert" doesn't agree with the world experts and may not even be aware of their view.

- To provide insight about how my privilege to practice medicine was cut away ["surgically"] from me in a way that I will show you was improper and unethical.

- To offer clear recommendations that could make college disciplinary processes more honest and fair, not just in my province but throughout Canada and the United States, at least.

- And to encourage those who find themselves in apparently hopeless situations, like the one in which I found myself, to not give in and give up, but live – even with emotional pain and challenges.

Knowing how this was done to me will give you insight about losses in general, and the vulnerability of every physician in Canada and the United States in particular. Your holocaust will probably differ from mine, but a few of you actually will have a challenge very similar to mine. Perhaps sanctions have already been taken against you, a colleague, or your doctor. Very often the public feels as though there were a black box in which the decision was made. Very often, the inexperienced feel that the black box must have proceeded rightly in whatever it did. That is a very self-reassuring viewpoint but incorrect.

So in order to help you understand the tormenting situation that my family has faced, I am going to bring experience to the inexperienced. The public needs a chance to see into the black box. Professional colleges have unfettered power and really need to use it appropriately, if the medical community and those patients who depend on them for medical care are to be safe. The alternative is a holocaust in which each person in trial needs a number of ways of coping in order just to survive. But that was my trial. Yours may be quite unrelated: cancer or career, diabetes or family abuse, an untenable work situation or divorce, accusations or other proceedings – any trial can wear you out, sap your energy, tax your resources. Frequently they make you doubt yourself or trusted others. They suck life from your family.

The quotations, regarding my trial, in this book are from letters in my possession, cited medical sources, the official transcripts from my "disciplinary hearing," or the official findings or written summaries from the panelists (tribunal judges) at my hearing. Here are my ground rules: I won't be telling you everything from the transcripts because they are fairly boring and too extensive; I will be completely accurate, but I will not specifically name the names of the offenders, much as they deserve to be shouted from the rooftops. I am doing this to avoid further quasi-legal proceedings from them. Also, because this subject is so dark in central theme (unethical behavior and the strain that brings individuals to consider suicide), I will attempt to use humor and references to motion pictures to lighten the grist. I have no wish to wear you out. I want to strengthen you, not weaken you. I do not want to do you harm.

I am going to talk frankly about how *being falsely accused of sexual assault can be quite similar to being sexually assaulted.* It makes you ask, "Why me?" It makes you ask, "Did I do something to bring this upon myself? Did I draw inappropriate attention to myself?" It suppresses your sexual interests and normal expression. It makes you feel guilty even if you rationally know that you aren't. It makes you have trust issues. It brings recurrent dreams and nightmares. It can be associated with or contribute to anxiety and depression. It makes you want to dress or look differently – so that you will not be recognized or noticed. You want to be invisible. It has left in me this posttraumatic residue. I am writing to enable my own healing, help others who suffer, and allow some accountability by those who bent rules to cause me harm, should they ever choose to become accountable. But I am also writing in celebration of those who helped me survive. I have not found any books that talk about this subject: only a few brief articles in magazines or journals. If there are any books, they are few and not well known.

A college may not be sued for taking an inappropriate disciplinary action. In this regard, the college is above the law: in fact, the college really IS the law! Wow! So as registrar, you may choose to behave as royalty of the past and say to one of the peons in your jurisdiction: "You have been weighed, you have been measured, and you have been found wanting. *In what WORLD could you possibly beat me?*" (Spoken by Count Adhemar in *A Knight's Tale*.) On the other hand, however, *an expert witness who misleads a disciplinary hearing committee* may be

1. *prosecuted* criminally for perjury,
2. *prosecuted* by her certifying organization, and
3. *prosecuted* civilly.

So why has she not been charged with perjury? I have been told that it is exceptionally rare for a charge of perjury to be pursued in Canada from a trial, let alone a professional hearing. But I am not a lawyer. So why am I not engaging one to pursue civil suit against her? Well, first and foremost, I don't really want to go back to the soul-sucking experience of legal wrangling. Secondly, I have, in fact, asked for a legal opinion from an experienced lawyer. He confirms that it is very difficult to sue an expert witness for negligence of her expert duties because you must be able to demonstrate that her dishonest, filtered evidence has caused a specific and quantifiable harm to your life. That is, that your life would have continued undamaged were it not for her misleading statements. It is one of the very premises of this book that the surgeon expert (of the two experts who testified at my hearing) was not the only "causer of harm" to my career, income, and life. It is true that I end up placing a lot of blame on the current registrar, who was the assistant registrar for my hearing and had been the chairman of the complaints committee earlier in the process. I also must blame at least one hearing committee member, my own liability insurance-assigned lawyer, and the investigator for the college. All these seem to have had a hand in my procedural assault.

It has been more than two years since the college erased me from the registry. This is about the time when I am able to grovel before the college and beg to be reinstated by them. I would be given very severe limitations and would have to publicly state that the college was completely right in how they proceeded. I would have to state that I had had sexual motivations for my "self-manufactured" methods of physical examination. I would have to show great remorse for having harmed those patients who made the *final four* complaints. This would directly infer that the complainants had been right and that I had been unfaithful to myself, my wife, and my profession. I cannot say that. It isn't true. I have been completely faithful to my training and my profession. I have been true to Dianne, my wife. I wouldn't be able to please the college with these facts. They are unlikely to reinstate me.

It is certainly uncommon for physicians to write about their conflicts with the College of Physicians and Surgeons of their province, state, or territory. This can be because they are burned out or emotionally crushed after a struggle that seems unwinnable: they are a small David against an insentient Goliath. It can be that they are struggling as Jonathan Livingstone Seagull because (almost) all of the gulls in the flock seem to have "turned their backs on" them. It can be because they fear further repercussions from that college. It can be because they feel that the college was right and proper in their dealings regarding them. And many colleges use a particular noose around their censured physicians' neck – with the implied threat that the noose can tighten at their slightest displeasure, but they are "allowed" to continue to practice, sometimes with very tight restrictions. For example, one college had an assistant registrar who seemed very understanding and compassionate. They unfortunately caught him embezzling funds from the college. He was required to publish a letter of contrition and subordination in that college's newsletter. Can you guess if they still have some power over him? This reprimanded ex-assistant registrar was called by the college to further testify against me in the proceedings based on the *final four* complainants (you'll note that I didn't call them the Fantastic Four even though the accusations by two of them were quite fantastic). Can you guess whether he used a tone and content that would please the existing college bureaucracy? A further alternative: a college can extend its control over a physician by limiting his or her practice – while still registering the physician and thereby keep him/ her "in line." Few physicians are willing to make public their feelings of having been wronged by the college while it still has this power over them. Only fellow physicians know, and this is usually by word of mouth – it is a gradually building and building group. After my first dealings with the "system," many other assailed physicians would make their way to my office wanting to talk. They needed to hear that their frustrations were legitimate from someone who would not condemn them.

In case you are unaware, let me emphasize that the medical association is not the College of Physicians and Surgeons in my province. The former has as its purpose to help all the doctors in the province. In theory, the latter is to protect the public: the citizens of the province. You may be insightful enough to realize that doctors would be some of the citizens of the province.

Honestly, we are all citizens and all patients. So while the association is known for helping doctors, the college should protect all patients, including those who happen to be doctors. I believe that has not been done in my case. Furthermore, the Canadian Medical Protective Association is a professional liability insurance company that exists to cover some of the costs of physician litigation. They, too, want to help. You are going to have the opportunity to decide who the good guys are – who wear the white hats. Are you ready?

CHAPTER I

THINGS TO KNOW ABOUT DOCTORS AND SURGEONS

A S EACH MEDICAL student has earned a place in a medical class, he or she has had to excel. That's how they got in. Usually, they were right more than those who were not chosen for admission. *Competition rules the admissions process.* In this regard, let me recount to you a true life experience. I was attending biochemistry class. Biochemistry is a subject mandatory for admission to medicine, in most schools. The lecturer presented a difficult subject one day. My study partner and I were confused by its complexity. However, the lecturer informed us that the subject was excellently presented in a text that was on reserve in the University of Calgary in the reference section. After the class, my friend and I sprinted to the library as rapidly as we could. Quickly we got to the library and its reference section. Imagine our dismay when the chapter in question had been razor-bladed out of the book! Competition! Beat the others! Make yourself look good or the others look bad! This competition is not over once you are admitted to a *traditional* medical school. You *compete for placement* in the class. To be number one or two in your class opens some real doors for your future. To be in the top ten is pretty heady.

If you are number 109 of 110, you will have trouble getting a job as a tollbooth operator. High ranking in your medical class will allow you to "choose your own adventure" in medicine – so *you MUST compete* [Rather like "You must get up, Bambi"]! However, in competing you won't necessarily have learned to work well with other doctors [similar to not being able to play well with other children]. Two universities in Canada have a different approach: Calgary and McMaster. I went to Calgary. There was no class placement specifically to foster working together, which we would hopefully do after medical school. Working together with other doctors has advantages to patients.

As we study within the medical faculty, we learn more the need to be RIGHT. Patients' lives depend on it! *We like to be right* for us. *We need to be right* for them! Sometimes we are very naïve in our belief that we are right. Sometimes we have the belief that the excellent way *we* were medically trained is the *ONLY* way to be medically trained: can any other method exist? It's like an obsession! We worship rightness [but perhaps . . . not righteousness].

Surgeons are a group of their own. They have a unique experience in medicine. Some believe that only the most arrogant miscreants choose to be surgeons, but this is not so! You must understand that there is not diagnostic certainty in some of the specialties – especially early in the process of helping a patient. Investigations are done and treatments are begun, and we see whether the hoped-for improvement occurs. The eventual amelioration proves that we were right, but it is not very immediate. This is not as often true in surgery. Surgery removes something or repairs something. It can remove, for example, an infected appendix. It can repair blood flow to heart muscle by bypassing an obstructed or narrowed passage. Arthroscopy can provide direct proof of a suspected condition. Subsequent surgery can completely replace the worn-out joint! Doing surgery very quickly confirms some diagnoses: we know pretty fast! It provides great affirmation that a problem has improved. It tells the surgeon that he/she was right! The affirmation comes pretty quickly. That provides those of us who have done surgery a fairly immediate *reward* in terms of feeling right, even powerful. It definitely contributes to our goal of being right. If some become arrogant after having repeatedly been affirmed, that is not too surprising.

CHAPTER 2

WHAT PAST MISTAKES HAVE I MADE
IN CLINICAL PRACTICE?

T HIS IS GOING to require a lot of personal disclosure. I need to supply the necessary background to my reading audience. I need to talk about my past experiences – that will be hard for me because after so many public disclosures *about me*, I became very private. I didn't want to tell anyone anything! Yet I am glad that you somehow acquired this book. I am glad that you are reading it because this is an important issue to medicine, to the law, and to the community. But I don't know you, most of you. And you don't really know me. *So much false information about me has been made public*, with part of the public treating it as irrefutable truth! Rather like the emptying of feathers from a pillow – the feathers can never be gathered up again, even the "wrong" feathers. I think at one time I used to be an extravert, but the experiences that I have gone through have made me very, very private. I have not disclosed things I didn't need to disclose . . . until now. Let me explain.

In my late teens and early twenties, I was very open. I wanted to learn everything, understand everything, and tell everything. I graduated from high school at age sixteen. I was an opinionated teenager, very unlike my own teens . . . NOT! I took stands. I was . . . a hippie, with a small *h*. In my youthful exuberance, I loved *CAUSES of fairness*. I liked public speaking. I loved telling or reading stories aloud. I loved the stage either as audience, chorus, or player. I enjoyed singing solo or with a choir. I enjoyed playing the violin: solo, accompanied, with a few others, or with an orchestra. I loved, in music, the blending of harmonies. I came to look forward to those precious moments in performance when a special chord or harmony would just blossom into our hearing. My mother had been a concert pianist before her family came. She would play for us in the dark – that bedazzled us. She taught us all to play the piano to start. Then, if we preferred, she allowed us to choose an instrument other than that at which she excelled. I chose the violin.

Mom also played the cello and was the first and only person we knew of to have a Solovox attached to the piano. This was an add-on electronic-amplified organ with which she would highlight her piano performances. It was called a Solovox for two reasons: It was made by the Solovox company (so just there is a pretty good reason), and although it had about twelve "stops" to allow various different sounds, it could only play one note at a time: Solovox=solo voice – no chords. For a skilled performer, however, its *accents* were very beautiful. I will always remember the big radio tubes in the amplifier. It looked very "advanced" at the time. It clipped onto the front of the piano, had big brown cables running to the amplifier, and had only about two and a half octaves of keys, and these keys were very small. It was the distant ancestor to the electronic keyboards of today, but I knew it from my youth. Familiarity with music in my home and performing with the family "band" made me willing to do what musicians do: *perform*! *Music is a performance art*, and all who really DO music must be willing to perform. Hence, I did violin solos at church, accompanied choirs and congregations, and once was on the Georgina Fooks Show on local Lethbridge, Alberta, television with the family band [even though our family didn't even own a TV 'til much later when I was fourteen and had moved to Calgary].

Music, public speaking, dance, and the theater taught us to be public, except about sex. Everyone in the late fifties and early sixties was private about sex. That was a part of why "Free Love" in the '60s became so popular. It seemed like it had been denied the growing generation. My mother taught us intimacy theory openly but taught us to be private [not secret] about it. She sometimes referred to a medical textbook that she had purchased. I think it must have been copyrighted about 1938 or so. Still, we learned the proper anatomic names for everything, very unlike many of our little friends from more embarrassed families. Because at my table we continued this tradition, my children laugh that a younger sibling complained that her "angina [not vagina] hurt" Angina is, of course, chest pain related to lacking oxygen. My later life trials taught me to be private about everything; well, everything personal, anyway. And I stopped being willing to perform music. Let me explain.

As every child, I had made some poor choices in life as I grew up. Nothing awful, but I was an imperfect teen. I became my version of a hippy. I thought I was involved in *"the movement of the 1960s,"* and I have never agreed with skin color superiority. But then I determined to study my own religion and found it to be honest, helpful, and sweet. I went on a mission for my church. Then I returned home and completed my bachelor's degree at the University of Calgary. I dated extensively and then met and married my wife, Dianne. She was gorgeous. She was musical. She believed, as I did, in family. She had stunning blue eyes (crowd stoppers), brunette hair, and a flawless complexion. She had the face of a model. She seemed like a fairy princess. I felt so lucky. We talked extensively about family planning because we planned to have a family. We later jokingly told others that we HAD to get married because we were expecting nine babies.

The morning after we were married, I had an interview at the University of Alberta through graduate studies with the department head in surgery, Tom Williams. He was such a gentleman and a scholar. Knowing him made me want to be like him. He was a fine leader and could mediate little squabbles gently and fairly. You may now ask, "What! Little squabbles in the department of surgery? How can that be? Surgeons are so educated and refined and honorable and gifted . . . and divine. How could a department full of them ever have squabbles?" But there were squabbles, and Tom calmed them. Perhaps their further training had made some of them think that their views were, in fact, NEVER WRONG. They had achieved the pinnacle of being right *all the time*. Tom knew better, but he was gentle. He introduced me to James Russell, a PhD chemist in the department, who was doing some research in renal preservation for transplantation. This was an extension of exactly what I had been doing in my last two years of undergraduate studies and what I had been doing for employment to support myself as a student. I had been a surgical technician to George Abouna, a transplant surgeon in Calgary. I had also worked in the lab at the Foothills Hospital. I was quite able to draw blood from pretty well any person, dog, rabbit, or mouse. I could take blood and start and pace IV drips before the fancy machines were available to control drip rates. I had fun doing this "medicine-support" work, and I was really good at IVs. I had very steady hands and acquired procedural skills very quickly. What it took three of us, initially, to do as a research team in two to three hours, I learned to do by myself in about forty-five minutes. These skills may be the reason that I was on George's transplant team when we did the first liver transplant in Western Canada on July 31, 1975.

FAMILY AND MEDICINE

Dianne became pregnant the month after we got married. We rejoiced in her pregnancy. She actually *cried and apologized* to me the previous month when she got a period. I so loved her that I would have accepted no children or many with her. But then, pregnancy was not easy for her. She got so much morning sickness that despite the (then) Bendectin (now, Diclectin), she had lost more than 10 percent of her body weight in the first trimester, by Christmas. Our dear family doctor, Peter Quandt, figured she'd need to be admitted to hospital for IV fluid therapy on our first Christmas Eve together. Not so nice. But then he relented and said, "Bryant, you're able to do this yourself at home, if you are willing." So on Christmas Eve, we picked up the supplies from the hospital and went to her parents' home. I hung the IV bag from the swag lamp in the room that had been hers previously and rehydrated her intravenously overnight, so that way, we could be together for our first Christmas. I so loved to be with her, any chance we got. And I came to both admire and love her wonderful parents.

We had that first baby; by bringing Rebecca Jo into the world, *Dianne made me a father.* I adored this baby girl and loved Dianne the more for having been the portal of this joy. We were in awe of this small life in our hands. I have to say also that that was the first time I saw a physician make a mistake. The intern who assisted in the delivery didn't know how to correctly hold a needle driver to stitch up the episiotomy that had (routinely) been done. He or she held the suture as if for a backhand pass and was clearly very awkward doing it. I volunteered, "You'll probably want to hold it so the needle points to the left"; that enabled a forehand pass. I think the young doctor was embarrassed that the father of the baby was telling him how the repair should be done. Remember premise 2? Uh-oh! That would mean he was wrong! But *this was my wife*!

The hospitals, then, made you feel like they were totally in *charge* of you – mother, baby, everything. They seemed to have rules for each situation. But then, *on the fifth day* when she was released from hospital, Dr. Quandt pushed her in a wheelchair to the ambulance bay doors where I had brought the car; she and the baby got in, and we closed the door. We were alone – just the three of us. I drove home very carefully. So then, there were no more rules, except the ones we made for ourselves. We chose what to do. We were a family. Nineteen months later, we had our first son, Michael Brandon. And our little Becky Jo loved him. She made room for him. She mothered him. Wow, my Litchfield name would continue in him! We felt so blessed. Dianne was able to cope with things. She was very organized. She made lists. She did most of the banking and shopping for us. She had so much energy. She prepared good food. She made it feasible for me to finish my graduate studies, write a master's thesis, and do a postgraduate year in computer science, statistics, astronomy, advanced physiology, and (for pleasure) violin performance while she finished her degree in education. We took that last class (violin) together. Wow! Was I lucky! I applied to medicine, dentistry, and law. I was admitted to law school at the University of Alberta in 1979. But while I was attending law school orientation week in Edmonton, the faculty of medicine in Calgary called and offered me a place in their medical class. Oh my! *I accepted immediately* on the phone, but then I had to talk with Dianne and ask what she thought, so we could "decide . . . together." Oops, my bad. She figured that medicine would be more of a commitment and forever take time from the family, and so she had been quite glad that I started with law (really law would have taken a lot of time too, to be good at it, but we were naïve). But she loved me and saw the light in my eyes come on when I talked of medicine. So she supported me, and we moved from Edmonton law school to Calgary medical school. Oh, miracle of miracles! I got in! I was joyful! But if I got in, then there were some other good men and women who really wanted to but did not get in. I had even had a close friend get in, finish, and then not intern. He had taken a place in the faculty of medicine, finished, and quit. He had his MD but went out internationally and bought and sold sulphur. Others did not get a place, and he took his and squandered it, I had thought. Well, as it turns out, I was wrong. He eventually came back and entered residency in OB/GYN. He now works in this field in Florida. I still have fond memories of him. I hope I have done honor to the place that I occupied in my medical class.

We had to borrow some money for school from that point on (I had no student loans up 'til then). So we carefully figured out what it would cost per month [Calgary was three years straight, rather than four academic years with summers off]. I asked for a loan of $6,900 for the year. We were told that it was clear that we needed the money, but the maximum we could get from student financing was $4,300. So we fretted in that first year of school – there was no time to work and earn money in breaks in the virtually year-round program. I was cautious in book purchases and borrowed a lot from the library: my little brown softcover textbook of physical examination, for example. I even went to talk with the Canadian military in late

September of that first of three years. Books and instruments were more expensive than we had planned for, and by January, we could see no way to do this without further assistance. So I went back to the military in January 1980 to talk mutual commitment. And I joined, as a junior officer (second lieutenant), making $700 per month. They paid me retroactively from September when I had first talked with them, and they paid for my instruments and books! We were rich! Well, *less poor anyway*, as every military man knows. We could see possibilities. We had Amy nine months later and Leisl eighteen months after Amy – four children before finishing medical school. Our personal happiness made our family grow. Our firstborn Rebecca happily introduced each new child to our family habits and rules; she was awesome, if eventually overburdened with being the "child leader."

After graduation, I accepted to intern at the Royal Jubilee Hospital in Victoria, British Columbia. It was a rotating internship in a hospital with almost no residents. We interns were it! We RAN the hospital . . . with a little help from the medical staff. Well . . . maybe more than a little help. But the staff really wanted us to become competent. And we learned to be exceptionally responsible. We did things correctly in the hospital, or patients suffered. I lived only about ten blocks from the hospital on Haltain Street. At a walk, I could be there in ten to twelve minutes, but at a run I could arrive very quickly; yet when we were on call for our medical service of the time, we had to sleep in the attached residence building; we each shared a room with another intern. If he weren't on call when I was, then I had the room to myself. But the truth is, we didn't sleep so much when we were on call because if there were a CODE, then the four of us on call all had to respond. Whoever got to the patient's room first coordinated the efforts of the others and made the final decisions, albeit listening to recommendations. It was about what you've seen on TV. And in spite of the weight of the responsibility, we learned to be sufficient. In that way I became like Dianne was: competent and self-reliant in my field.

I had never been to Victoria before. It is such a beautiful city, on such a beautiful island. But I was there for internship, not tourism, so I never toured the sights. Dianne would take the children places and make life fun for them. She taught little Becky how to walk to kindergarten at the "big girl" school. I was only home some of the time, but at least then, my hours were sort of predictable, and we were better paid because I was promoted in the military to first lieutenant. The internship programs loved to get us military guys because they didn't have to pay us from their internship program budgets. The year went smoothly. I learned more about gynecology from three lady doctors there who shared their two practices with me than I had possibly imagined before. I was the doctor who coordinated interns working at the birth control clinic in Victoria. I wanted to do this because I felt I didn't, even then, know much about women. And I didn't. My wife will attest to that. Maybe she would even now.

So I learned lots more about women's health, and in recompense, these three doctors provided huge experience to me. One of them offered to teach me how to do abortions. That was very hard for me to consider. I declined, respectfully. First, I had a *strong Christian faith* that specifically was opposed to unnecessary abortion. Second, I had learned in school this *profound respect for all life* and my duty to preserve it. One windy gray day, she paged me to provide a surgical assist to her in performing a midtrimester abortion to a psychiatric, street drug–using patient. This procedure may have been warranted. I prayed as I walked over to the hospital and operating room. But I did my "intern duty" and scrubbed with her. I was in anguish. I was told that even if the baby were born alive, it could not survive, and we were *not to attempt* to resuscitate or sustain it. As we did the C-section, it became apparent that the baby had actually died sometime previously, as the little body was already decaying. I felt sad for that little body, but I was so grateful that I had not put my skills to the ending of its life, nor had had to withhold my skills if it should be born alive. I never since have directly participated. I know several of my patients have made those choices, but neither am I condemnatory of them because that, too, is not my profession nor my faith. In fact, with a later patient who was struggling to make a good decision for herself, her quandary was on my mind most of the time. I wrote at that time the following poem:

Reflexions on Abortion: I almost Threw You Away

I almost threw you away.

I throw away old
Cabbages, or dry bread with mould.
I throw away worn shirts,
Or old paint pants holed.

I almost threw you away.

I almost threw you away. Almost
Missed the dimples in your hands and in your face:
Take first steps . . . sit back down hard, make my knee your space.

I almost threw you away . . . almost I threw you away:
I wanted to think of you as a pouch of mush, somehow.
No eyes, no ears, no hands, no beating heart . . . not now.

I almost gave away my chance for you to stay.
For me to share . . . my language while I watch you play.
Introduce your friends – help you tie up loose ends;
Teach you thank you and please . . . until you wanted my . . . keys.

I almost threw you away . . . really, I almost threw you away – 'cause
There've been so many times I've thought someone should throw
Me away too.

I finished my year of internship and hoped to be posted up island
to a most isolated base at Holberg. That didn't happen. I was sent to
CFB Borden – not at all isolated. I did my basic training there too. God
bless the sergeants and warrant officers who took us through basic.
They certainly had their work cut out for them 'cause remember we
were doctors and captains who both like to be right. As captains, we
outranked them, but we sure didn't know much military stuff. One
day I came to classes and my chief (warrant officer) noticed that I was

wearing my own slightly wider (and much prettier) belt. He took me aside and "ripped up one side of me and down the other." He yelled, "What, Litchfield, have you joined a motorcycle gang?" The honest truth is, he had committed his whole life to this honorable profession, and he had little time for any who were just waterskiing behind him. *Had we no honor?* I determined that I would live my military/medical life with honor.

The promotion to captain included a significant raise in pay. We lived on the base on Sangro Loop with a bunch of other junior officers. The dad of the family next door introduced himself as a spy, really. Each Saturday morning, we were awakened by cannon and tank fire on the range. There were nine or ten painted tanks in the park near our house for the children to play on. My wife actually became the president of the Officers' Wives Club in Borden the second year we were there. She was very friendly and very organized. They loved her. I loved her. Becky and Michael started kindergarten and prekindergarten in Borden, and Amy at age three bravely got dressed and caught the school bus to preschool every day. Becky and Michael walked her each time to her pick-up and drop-off site near their school. I so loved that they cared for each other. And I began to get those strong protective instincts of fatherhood. I wanted them each to be included by others and happy in their blossoming lives. Dianne and I were really happy, and so, of course, we had our fifth child (Shawn) there. We became part of the military community in Borden and part of the religious community in Barrie. Life was good.

I was still naïve about some things. It always took me longer to see patients than the other junior medical officers. We did sick parade in the mornings and did three medicals in the afternoons. Then we could go home. Some, starting at 1:00 p.m. could finish their "medicals" by 1:50 p.m. (about fifteen minutes per "complete" medical). The military support staff loved that; they liked us to work briskly. I think it was called sick parade because they wanted to keep the sick marching . . . or at least, moving – even through our offices. I was still fairly slow and analytical. I simply believed what I had been taught about possible pathology. So I took my time. And

I really searched for problems. What obsessive-compulsive traits I naturally had, medical training had increased. I knew each night when I went to bed, though, that I had done my best, and so I could sleep well.

The base surgeon made up specific areas of responsibility for each of the junior medical officers. I didn't much like my first base surgeon. He had not remembered much medicine. He was administrative. He was political. He didn't take "call" on the base, thankfully. I began moonlighting in a rural hospital emergency room in Alliston, off base, to keep my skills keen. The deputy base surgeon had a farm in the vicinity and clearly was biding his time with the military and with medicine. He proudly proclaimed that he hadn't "cracked a book or journal" in his fourteen years in the military medical corps since graduation in medicine at the U of A. I questioned the base surgeon about his capability to run a code if that should come up while it was his turn to be on call. I was firmly told that criticizing a superior officer "doesn't go" in the military.

I did find some comradeship with the other two junior medical officers though: Kim Williams and Andy McCallum [I am using their actual names – with fondness]. They had trained together in Toronto. Kim had developed a romance in medical school with another student, married, and then divorced him. Medical school romances so often seemed to fail, but they were common. It has something to do with coming of age sexually. While she was posted in Borden, she had a relationship with a successful businessman in the nearby little town of Angus. The base surgeon became aware of this and told her several times that she should not have that relationship because it was not *conduct becoming* an officer. She and I didn't consider him a very good judge of appropriate conduct: he did not have a healthy body or habits, for a physician. I felt sorry for Kim, and I commiserated with her about how the peacetime military worked. More recently, Canada has again required a wartime military. A significant number of our service personnel have been killed. That changes everything. A doctor in the Canadian forces now would be deployed to battle zones with his/her regiment. Not so when I served. Now, some give the ultimate sacrifice, and many come away with *having seen too much and having something broken inside.* I have such respect for them. I pray for them.

I must have made myself disliked by my base surgeon. [Note here that this person in power figured that *conduct unbecoming* an officer was pretty well anything he said it was. I think we'll see this same thing in MY story.] Because it was popular and new and energetic, I hoped to be made responsible for sports medicine for the base. That would be a feather in my cap, I thought. I was really let down when he made me responsible for the "hole in the ground" (communication and support in case of nuclear, biological, or chemical crisis) and for drug and alcohol rehabilitation for Base Borden. "But, sir," I argued, "I am the only junior medical officer on the base who has a family. In a crisis I would want to be with them. And I don't know anything about drug and alcohol use, let alone rehab, because I don't ever drink alcohol."

"Litchfield" he said, "orders are not open to discussion." Even now it sounds so very military, doesn't it? Some things really did "go" in the military.

LEARNING TO BE A COUNSELOR

So I became tasked with those duties. In addition, during basic training, I was required to qualify with a nine-millimeter handgun on the range. I was told that if I was duty officer on some base one night, a sidearm was a part of my uniform. I was encouraged to become proficient with it because I might be faced sometime in the future with an enemy who would try to steal medical supplies, and *then what would I do?* "Well, I'd let him have them," I thought to myself. I didn't really have much killer instinct left in me. My hunting days were over. I respected wildlife as all other life, now. I have no idea how I would have functioned in a wartime military.

But at that time, I had to learn about alcohol and drugs. Why would those be a particular problem in the military? As it turned out, it was a problem. The enlisted men and women were very young, away from home, making all their personal decisions on their own and perhaps reckless. Their duty hours were pretty strictly dictated and controlled. But after duty, or on leave, they could buy *subsidized booze* at the junior ranks mess. And some of them, even in a nonwartime era, loved to lose themselves in alcohol. And with the subsidization they figured the military kind of approved of drinking; it was even a ceremonial part of mess dinners. [This has always been perplexing to me.] I was sent in 1984 on a perhaps six-week course to Long Beach, California, with the US Navy to learn about the extent and nature of the problem and to start to comprehend approaches to its resolution. I learned about AA and Al-Anon, NA and Narc-Anon and addictive gambling, sex, and eating addictions. There could well be a twelve-step program now for addiction to video games or violence, as I have seen these become addictive to some. Pornography certainly can be. The key isn't simply *time given to the pursuit*; it's whether *relationships with living people* (as opposed to virtual ones) *have been harmed* as a result. If you have an addiction, then you know inside what I mean. I continued the interest I had developed as an intern, in anorexia and bulimia, which may involve a media-mediated addiction to the concept of thinness. I became a friend to AA and have regularly attended some of their open meetings for the twenty-five years since then. The great humility that it takes to twelve-step progress along the road to recovery put me in awe. It still does now.

Therefore, early in my medical practice years, I started really listening to people and considering alcohol health issues: what they said in words and what they conveyed in other ways. That didn't speed me up in doing my office duties. I was very methodical. I guess I started thinking holistically. I remember so clearly doing a medical one afternoon on a man who had had four other medicals within the previous year. "What schlock!" I thought. He had been promoted to corporal, reup'd [reenrolled in the military after a contracted time had been served], been posted overseas for three months, and returned from that posting, and now was being promoted again, to sergeant this time. Each required a complete medical. Now it was my turn to do his fifth in one year. Wow, what a waste of time! But I'm obsessive, and I know about duty. So I went through the thing, exactly the way I have been trained. When we got to the part of the physical exam where I do a genital and rectal exam on a man, I asked,

"You've never had a significant lump or mass in the scrotum, right?" And he said, as he slipped down his underwear, "No, never!" But he had one: a firm, nontransilluminating [I could not pass light through it] eleven centimeters (three and a half inches in diameter) mass in his left testicle space. Oh gosh, I thought, but I said, "You're kidding me, right?"

I knew this would be almost certain cancer, and I felt sick. I said, "Look, Sarge, how can this be? You've had four other medicals this year." "Yeah," he said, "but *you're the first one who ever actually checked me.*" I quickly arranged for him to be seen at Sunnybrook Hospital in Toronto the next day. He had three kinds of cancer in that mass, and at least one type had already spread (metastasized). He had the testicle removed that day and was on chemo by the end of the week. I will never forget that exchange: it came early in my career, and it came with power. Pathology does exist! I had taken an oath when I became a physician, and I resolved, again, to keep it forever. I have.

MAKING MYSELF VULNERABLE

Also at Borden, a young corporal in the records department asked me to see an acquaintance of hers who had been raped on an isolated base on Vancouver Island. She said it was complex and would take some time, so I allowed that she book it through the front desk. The young lady came in to my office. I had never dealt with rape before, on my own, but my internship had taught me to be "sufficient." Having been forewarned of her plight, I sympathetically pulled my chair over to her side of the desk and sat directly in front of her. I thought that was a good start. I took notes in her temporary file as we talked. She was in Borden, as many military were, on course. That means she came from her base to ours for some kind of training. She recounted a dreadful story. On her base on Vancouver Island (just up island from where I had recently lived), there was not much to do in your time off. In the mess for enlisted persons, with the alcohol being very cheap, she (with her acquaintances) had consumed too much. They were dancing and drinking, drinking and dancing. She finally went back to her barracks and crashed in her room to sleep it off. Apparently, one of the fellows who had danced with her had wanted more. He followed her back to her barracks and waited for her to sleep. He then had entered her room, removed her clothing, raped her, and left her naked in her bed. When she had wakened the next day and found herself naked in bed, she had no idea what had happened. Over the days that followed, she became aware of jokes that were being told about her, and she deduced that she had been raped. She became the brunt of a lot of ill humor.

I was shocked and saddened by her story. I asked if she had been seen by the medical people and military police at her base. She said that she had, but by the time she had been seen, for the assault, she had had consenting sex with at least a couple of other men. The medical people had done swabs for infectious diseases but could apparently offer little else, at that point. And she did not actually remember any of the rape sequence: perhaps a blessing but also hard to try to describe to the police. There seemed nothing that she could do. As she described her situation, it became clear that she was more upset by the ridicule than by the unchosen sex. So I was left with a young woman who was angry about the ridicule but had no ongoing problems with intimacy. In fact, I wonder if I conveyed that she might have been a little liberal in her consenting sex life. The experience had not made her uncertain about sex or herself; it just made her angry over being made fun of. She didn't consider her alcohol use a problem. She continued to drink and "party" in her off-duty hours.

I, too, could not really provide her justice for the way she had been abused. I had no administrative power to investigate her complaint against her fellow soldier, being simply a doctor at a distant base. I probed about her alcohol use though because that was my "special" duty. I asked if she had had any other blackouts after drinking. I tried to help her see that of the things we could still now deal with, the way that she used alcohol might be among the most important. I think that made her angrier, not at some vague fellow soldier, but at me.

I had still been compulsively reading medical books and journals regularly and had recently come across an article that commented on chest telangiectases (spider nevi – these are little surface veins rather in the shape of the spokes of an umbrella) in consequence of heavy alcohol consumption. I asked that she unbutton the top of her shirt to show the V of skin in front of the sternum area. She did this, and I actually did find two or three spider nevi [but I didn't really know if that meant there WAS a big problem]. Perhaps she saw my request as an order, and I certainly did outrank her because I was an officer. If this is the case, then I am sorry for the implications. It is possible that she would not have willingly unbuttoned her shirt before a male doctor outside of the military. I may have been a power figure to her, but I thought of myself as her servant, a helper. I have always thought of myself in my capacity as a doctor – not as having *power over others*, but as having *power with others*: what power I have is by working *with* my patient.

My journal article had only alerted me to the *possibility* of that clinical sign. She wasn't very old but had been drinking already significant volumes of alcohol for a few years. She claimed she could generally "hold" her liquor. Nonetheless, this drinking had led to a problem for her [it had rendered her defenseless and amnesic], and one of the working definitions of alcoholism was the continuation of drinking behavior when it had caused a major problem previously (like causing an accident with injury while driving under the influence). I asked her to book a complete medical so that I could make us both aware of her health and determine any medical consequences of excessive alcohol. I can see, in retrospect, that I occupied a position of authority. I was a medical officer requiring an enlisted person to come for an appointment. She apparently resented me, and she had some real emotional baggage. My position of authority also made me vulnerable to her situation. And she lashed out.

ACCUSED, INTERROGATED, BUT NEVER CHARGED

Instead of seeing her the next week, I was interrogated by the military police. It seems she had lodged a complaint through channels. She took all of the anger she had stored up from the rape and ridicule and focused it at me. The military police on *my* base DID become involved, deeply. I spent hours in interrogation with various MPs. It was almost surreal. Oh my goodness! She talked a friend into also making a complaint, and the story just got bigger and bigger on the base [which is so very much like a very small town where everyone knows everything about everyone else]: scandal is the very lifeblood of gossip. [Hence, the recent so sad news from Trenton, Ontario, concerning their base commander accused of rape and murder]. The most common accusation about me was that in the course of some kind of office medical contact, I had made someone "feel uncomfortable" – one, during an eye exam. I had been "a subject" talked about in the junior ranks mess. The accusations were entirely lacking any aspects of physical assault or sexual arousal on my part or theirs, they acknowledged. They were more "just a feeling I got" type accusations, but I did get lots of this stressful interrogation time with the various military police, one of whom questioned his own girlfriend closely and then she made a complaint. This might be called a cascade or domino effect. Although I was then registered with the College of Physicians and Surgeons of Ontario, the military preferred to keep things in-house. And *they really know how to interrogate.* That was a stressful time. However, the complaints were never published. I made my wife aware, but our children were able to remain blissfully unaware. I suppose that my conversation with that original enlisted person MIGHT have made her uncomfortable because it reminded her of her ridicule and embarrassment, but I had thought I was just "doing my duty."

In the end, I was neither charged nor arrested. I was spoken to by the base surgeon, the base commander, and finally the chief surgeon for the Canadian forces. He said, "Use a chaperone to *protect YOURSELF!*" Even after this, one prior patient, who had moved to another base, blackmailed me with a threat of making a similar complaint against me, from a distance. "Do you want to go through all that stuff again?" she asked me on the phone. Obviously things weren't kept entirely in-house. She wanted $20,000: some easy money. I invited her to come and talk with my wife and I in Borden. Then I myself went to the military police about the blackmail. No charges were ever laid against either of us. Well, it *was* kept in-house . . . sort of.

During the investigation, I had kept busy lecturing at the school for TQ6 medics and teaching them how to respond to emergencies. Then I had resumed my work as a junior medical officer. The new base surgeon asked me to counsel a new junior medical officer about similar matters. And I still did my moonlighting at the Alliston Hospital near CFB Borden. The president of the medical staff there, a woman, talked with me about my report to her about the accusations. She was so very understanding and supportive. She described a few of the complaints that had been made about her over her years of doing internal medicine. She said she'd once been complained of to the college for telling a younger female patient to not worry about her breast size because she had "very nice little boobies." I made a mental note to never walk that path by commenting on body parts. Without that shared experience, who knows, I might have thought that "being a guy" I could compliment a woman from my "neutral" medical position. I recall my mom telling us at the dinner table that her doctor had just complimented her on her "trim figure" after her medical. That was obviously a faux pas by today's standards. Not everyone considers doctors to occupy a neutral position. Be really careful, my colleagues.

My dear wife, Dianne, still the president of the Base Borden Officers' Wives Club, was pregnant for the sixth time. And this time things were complicated. Becky, Michael, Amy, and even toddler Leisl understood that there was a problem with their mom. Baby Shawn just kept being a very dear boy – I worried for him as he grew that he was so naïve and dear that someone might take advantage of him. But at this time he was a precious baby, and his mom had bleeding from a central placenta previa. That means that the placenta is blocking the exit from the uterus (the cervix) so that the baby could not possibly be born via normal labor. Small pullings away of the placenta from the uterine wall to accommodate the growing baby resulted in little bleeds. She was first on bed rest at home, and then on bed rest at the Barrie Hospital, and then sent to a major Toronto hospital. Her first bleed was at twenty-two weeks, and she was on bed rest in hospital after her second bleed at twenty-four weeks. Gradually, with help at home with my five children from my mother (who had thought of herself as too old to help such a young family), we got to thirty weeks. God bless my mother who always wanted to be a midwife to enable the gentle passage from God's arms to ours.

SURGICAL RESIDENCY

I had always been very involved in surgery and had been interviewed for that residency program at Dalhousie. Once again, I was sought after because I had a strong background in surgery and because the program could afford to have me in addition to any others because they didn't have to pay me. I was still paid by the military. The military was willing that I give my final required year of service as a surgical resident. What a gift! But I was required to move myself and my family to Halifax with Dianne in hospital in Toronto. After saying a tearful and frightened good-bye to her at the Women's College Hospital with my five children and mother, I departed. Our local family doctor at the time, Brian Morris, with whom I did medical journal club in Barrie, travelled from Barrie to Toronto a couple of times to see Dianne and reassure her. What a fine example. I wanted to be like Brian Morris. He was our hero and friend as well as Dianne's doctor. He was very involved in his patients' families – a true family doctor.

I wasn't able to be with Dianne for David's delivery. I was travelling to Nova Scotia to my new posting and stopped for the night in Montreal. Once my mother and I had bedded the five down in our motel for the night, I went out to an outdoor pay phone and called to check on Dianne. They actually wheeled her stretcher out to the hospital unit desk so that I could talk with her. While we were on the phone together talking, her voice turned to panic as she suddenly bled again hugely and was rushed down the hall into emergency surgery. The phone picked up the bustle for a while, and then was hung up. I was in panic mode. When I called again, I was informed that she was unavailable as she was in surgery. Sleepless hours later, when I called, I was told that the surgery was over and that Dianne was safe. I was told she could tell me about our baby when she was less groggy.

The next day she told me about our tiny David, just over four pounds. Those phone calls in separation became like reaching through the lines to her and David with my hands, my ears, and my heart. When he had stabilized somewhat medically, he and Dianne were later airlifted by the military to Halifax to continue his care at the Isaak Walton Killam Hospital where I was working as a surgical resident. When I finished my surgical resident duties each day, I would go up to his floor and just hold his precious little premie body and rock him. He liked to suck the tip of my thumb, so sometimes with his gentle rhythmic sucking of my thumb, he would fall asleep, and so would I. I guess the nurses took some pictures of us. He lives today with his wife and their baby boy in Saskatoon, where he studies also to become a doctor. My second base surgeon, Lt. Col. McKenzie, actually knit him an afghan attached to a baby blanket. It was such beautiful work and such a thoughtful gesture on her behalf. Kudos to you, Ruth McKenzie, *you weren't just military*!

So my final year in the military was as a first year surgical resident through Dalhousie. I loved doing surgery, and I loved studying the journals and texts that were associated with residency there. However, my wife and I had now had six children, and I had delivered a lot of babies, as a medical student and an intern. I just couldn't give up my main love – obstetrics and pediatrics (pregnant moms and their babies/children). Only family medicine would let me do both. So when that year was finished, in Halifax, we came back to Dianne's hometown – Edmonton – to do family medicine. Her wonderful parents were here, and our children were growing to love them because Grandpa let them join him "to fix stuff" and go boating and Grandma made these amazing head-of-state dinners served on plates that looked expensive. When we went to Grandma's house, Dianne would remind them, "Restaurant manners." Dianne's mom taught me how to waterski. They were "way good vacationers," my in-laws, maybe because they were both schoolteachers and had time off in the summer.

Because I had only delivered a pair of twins in a snowstorm during my three years in the military and residency, I took three months off my group practice at the end of 1987 and three months at the beginning of 1988 to update in obstetrics and pediatrics, respectively. I delivered hundreds more babies in Medicine Hat because of the willingness of the family medical doctors and two obstetricians there. I became confidant. Then I did a pediatric residency block at the University of Alberta Hospital. I became the first doctor in seven years to be given family practice obstetrical privileges at the Royal Alexandra Hospital. No one else at the Europa Medical Centre wanted to do hospital medicine: maybe I would do obstetrics for our whole group?!

NEW ORDERS, ALBEIT NONMILITARY

Then my senior partner at Europa clinic came to me one day and just said, "Bryant, you can't use our nurse as a chaperone for all your exams. Women don't really like it, and you're *monopolizing* her time." He just cut me off. Oh dear, that would make me more vulnerable. He didn't want to discuss it. Like being in the military! And *I LET HIM ORDER ME*! How I regret that. "Well," I reasoned, "this isn't the small town feeling of Base Borden anymore with tons of young people drinking and carousing each night. It might be safe. There isn't a natural officer-hate against me here, and he is my "boss." I guess . . . I'll compromise and abide his decision [since he didn't really give me any choice]." I have only realized, now long after, that *my use of a chaperone might make his nonuse of chaperones more noticed* or suspect; sort of like, if you do things more thoroughly than others, it might *seem like* they are not doing enough. But I did comply.

So the patients whom I then continued to see at Europa Medical Centre (who then eventually transferred with me to my new private office) became used to being unattended by a chaperone. I think they probably did prefer it. But I was unprotected; I had no one to vouch for me if someone complained. Furthermore, in the midspring of 1988, this senior partner went "on holiday" for a month. He went to Vancouver and bought two sailboats for occasional personal use and for investment as rental vessels. He had really learned how to make medicine pay. He could see sixty to eighty patients during his seven – to eight-hour shifts. I didn't know how he did it. I did know he would stack his charts on his desk during the week and come in on the weekend with a bottle of wine and write his notes in the four to five hundred charts! I was far too obsessive to consider doing anything like that: what might I forget? *What did he forget?*

Once again, the support staff of that clinic pressed me to go *faster*, see patients *quicker*, (rise *higher*), and get a greater patient volume through the till ASAP [the rise higher, not really to become an Olympian, but because now the clinic was getting PAID 40 percent of what I billed, so schlock 'em through Dr. B]. We didn't see eye to eye on how medicine should be done, my senior partner and I. And I guess also on many other aspects of life. He had been twice married and divorced. He was glitzy. He loved to drink. He had relationships with many of the female office staff and married our "head nurse" eventually. He became a friend to a surgeon, the man who became the registrar. Dr. RE was a party guy; maybe his new friend was too?

MY FORMER PARTNER

It was during his "junket" to Vancouver that a pharmacist called me and asked me to authorize a prescription that this partner had written. Why would I need to do that? I learned from the pharmacist over the phone that this senior partner had been *suspended from medical practice* by the college for a month. I was completely pole-axed. *HE had not informed me* of his suspension; he had just left "on holiday"! My other senior partner was having some health issues; maybe she fretted that she, too, couldn't do medicine as fast as this partner wanted. So mostly, I was the remaining senior person left to carry the practice. And when I asked the staff to provide me contact information for that partner at his vacation location in Vancouver, I found that *he had refused*. He cowardly assigned one of our nurses, Pam DeLuca [I *totally* wanted to provide her name 'cause she was great] to "just inform me" of his issues. He later fired her. It was only through her that I learned of his suspension for having questionably consensual sex with a patient whom he had been counseling at an office *in his home*! The real issue is, *can ANY needy patient actually give informed consent* to have sex with her medical helper? Was I able to trust him and leave my patients in his care when I was away? It was then that I felt I could no longer work under his "seniorness." So I informed him of my decision to leave the practice, found a place, and built a small solo-practice office across the hall from my friend and confidant, Dr. Doug Armstrong. I didn't really want to go from one partnership to an uncertain other one, so I went out as a solo practitioner. I had to invest a lot to do this, but I felt that I really could not trust that partner, with my patients, so there was no other way. The other senior partner and one of our associates like myself also left him and opened their own office. In fact, I let them use my new office in the evenings and weekends 'til they could have theirs built. I heard, later, that that senior partner resented <u>me</u> for *wrecking his practice.* How ironic! He took advantage of his vulnerable patient yet felt it was I who wrecked his practice. More ironic was that the College of Physicians and Surgeons of Alberta only suspended HIM for one month! With no damaging publicity! A slap on the wrist! A chance to invest in a fleet! He located elsewhere with another of the clinic doctors and then eventually went to the USA with our clinic's head nurse. That marriage too failed. Three for three! Wow!

I opened my office at Meadowlark Professional building, and I hired our nurse, Pam DeLuca, to *come back to work – with me*! I was across the hall from the Armstrong's and just down the hallway from the fine pair of surgeons, Dave Adams and Trevor Theman. I certainly referred anything surgical to Dave and Trevor even though I was now on staff not at their hospital but at the Royal Alexandra Hospital. I had nothing but satisfaction from those patients I sent to Dave or Trevor. I found that if I had a surgical challenge, being good neighbors, they would talk with me on the phone easily and occasionally see a patient from my office just minutes after I called. Wow, what a fine relationship we had! In addition, I began to do part-time maternity leave for their hospital, the Misericordias's staff physician (wondering if I might be able to transfer privileges to the Misericordia Hospital, which was much closer to home and to the office).

Life was good. I was happy. In February of 1987, we had had Cameron, and in June of 1989, we had Marcus (our eighth baby).

We had eight children! There was a show on TV called *Eight is Enough*. We shopped in wholesale places. You had to have a business in order to get a wholesale card back then. My medical office/business got me the card easily, but it bugged me that without me, Dianne could not get a card. She had her degree in teaching [early childhood – appropriate, huh?] for heaven's sake! So I applied for a separate card for her. Where the form came to listing her occupation, I wrote that she was the *director of a Home for Gifted Children* (mine). They gave her a card immediately. We loved our own pregnancies, and I loved helping others with theirs. I had found my niche. Although I did attend older patients also, I *just loved maternity care*. And I had had good role models for doing it: Peter Quandt, Yosh Okamura, Brian Morris, and many doctors in Medicine Hat, Alberta (like Peter Best) to name a few.

But remember how I said that the patients who came with me from Europa to my new office were used to seeing me unchaperoned. Well, now I had a new office and I could make my own rules, but I was swayed by our new habit of no chaperones. It was what our transferring patients had become used to, and I really could not afford to hire more than one person to work with me. Someone had to answer the phones, I figured. So I used the staff person only for procedures like minor surgery and IUD placement. *I will always regret that decision* to keep doing things the way I had been compelled to at the Europa clinic. So eventually something happened for which I would really have liked to have had a chaperone present.

NEED FOR A CHAPERONE

It was July 1989, Marcus was less than two months old. Oh, how I loved to see him in the crib in our closet as I would go through in the morning to shave in our washroom and dress for work. He was always so happy. He would let me pick him up and snuggle him, and then lie him back down again without a cry. That allowed me to not waken his mother as I left for work. Dianne and I were parents of eight beautiful children. Rebecca Jo was twelve, Michael was ten, Amy was turning nine, Leisl was seven, Shawn was turning six, David was four, Cameron was two and a half, and Marcus less than two months. Each of them had great sweetness; each was so individual. No two could be treated the same. It wasn't a group thing to raise eight children; each required his or her own time and approach. Five boys and three girls. And we were fortunate enough to know a few other large families then and got to know more such families since. I was a protective dad. If a daughter didn't feel popular or attractive, I suffered with her and tried to help as far as a dad can. I remembered times when I had not felt included growing up younger/smaller than all my schoolmates. If a son wanted to stand on his head, I tried to learn how to stand on mine. I shared imaginary stories with my children and occasionally with their cousins. We hosted original karaoke parties in our home because we were comfortable performing in public. The mother of my children was an amazing and assertive woman. If the school said they were allocated to such and such a class without their friends, I would volunteer to talk to the school. And they would say to me, "Dad, thanks for your willingness, but could you have Mom call – you're too nice on the phone. Mom gets things done!" But they had started to look out for each other too! The older ones each had a younger roommate. I think we were at peace.

On Wednesday July 24, 1989, I attended a young woman who complained of left-sided abdominal pain, right-sided low back pain, and constipation. During my exam, I noted that she had a redundant portion of sigmoid colon, and that portion (as far as I could feel on rectal and vaginal exam) was full of pelletlike stool. I discovered that there really wasn't a need to do a rectal exam on a person on whom pelletlike (not the usual sausage and soft) hard stool had been discovered in the course of the pelvic exam. Those pellets made diagnosis of the other complaints difficult while the diagnosis of constipation was obvious. I suggested that we have her use laxatives for a few days and then do a follow-up appointment. But she phoned two days later and requested an *urgent* reappointment because she was feeling worse and had been *UNABLE to work*. I asked my staff to add her on to the end of our patient load that day. I had a lengthy counseling appointment booked as my last patient, so resaw this add-on before that session, thinking it might easily be disposed of, perhaps with an urgent surgical referral. She had apparently taken some laxatives and moved a little stool, but the reexam showed no real change: there was still a lot of constipation.

OK, so this wasn't going to be quick. I had my nurse *go out and buy* two Fleet enemas and administer them to this patient, asking that she require the young lady to hold them as long as humanly possible (When you receive an enema, it often causes a fairly immediate strong urge for a bowel movement. However, if the enema is quickly evacuated, it will be less effective. Hence the need to wait even for a half hour all the while feeling a very strong urge to poop).

I, in the meantime, went back to my counseling patient who was a profoundly obese but emotionally immature adult. I can recall nothing of what I talked of with her that particular day, but I know that I saw her because with my appointment book and my charts I was able to reconstruct quite a bit of this scenario. This is more than twenty years ago, but I remember this disabled patient very well. I continued to attend her for a long time until her profound obesity and her mental inability to control her own food intake required her to be admitted to the hospital, and then extended care. That night when I finished my counseling session with her, I went back to the postenema patient.

My lawyer informs me that this constipated young woman in question had come to the office wearing very short shorts and had been reading a romance novel in my waiting room. He says she may have come intentionally looking very attractive, ready to flirt. He tells me she may have *intended to attract me.* I don't know. I wasn't ever good at telling those things after I was married (maybe even before). Dianne would occasionally enlighten me about what feminine flirting behaviors were. Further, I don't really try to notice what people wear to my office unless a senior citizen has had her hair done and is wearing dressy clothes. Then, I think, *I may be the only one who has noticed,* and I warmly compliment her. Does any elderly person get too many compliments? Except in that instance, I will *never* comment on clothing. My chief of staff in Alliston had made her point. How pretty her eyes are, how full his lips, how muscular he seems, how curvaceous she is, and any kind of underwear cannot draw my comment. That is not my business. Health is my business, and *I would comment on how healthy a patient looks*. I also comment on tans because UV light exposure is my business: I need to encourage moderation.

In any case, I did not see her when she came into the waiting room area anyway. So I have no idea how handsome she may have looked. I did recall that when she had come in two days before, she was with a reasonably healthy-looking young man. I thought they were a couple. I don't recall him well, but I usually made note of apparent couple mismatches, and I would only remember if the mismatch was striking. I figured that he was probably out there waiting for her this time too. My lawyer says he wasn't, but I didn't know that. It may be that she came in dressed in a way that she figured would draw the gaze of any man. But I first saw her that second day, undressed below the waist with a paper sheet over her lower half, having just had very effective bowel movements after a double enema. Forgive my bluntness, but this is hardly a romantic setting. Surely, recent bowel movements are not an aphrodisiac to anyone . . . well, maybe to some very strange fraternities in California. At some point the disabled woman with whom I had been counseling, and who often would finish reading an article in the waiting room that she had started, left the office area, and *my nurse came and said she was leaving* for the night. That left me alone. Oh, our naivety in those days. But on with my account.

I reexamined her pelvis and found that the stool was appropriately gone but discovered a large left ovarian mass: *two to three inches in size*. At least part of the mass felt cystic. A problem! I was worried. Now my mind was in overdrive – the worst possible case scenario would be a solid left ovarian tumor with a cystic component. There clearly was some significant kind of pathology here. Now what other facts did I have to work with? Left lower quadrant abdominal pain, constipation, and right lower back pain. Poop. Back pain. In primary care medical practice, headaches and back pain are perhaps the two most common chronic (ongoing) complaints – and the worst taught in medical school. No real logical process-of-exclusion approach was ever taught about these subjects. So the family doc with no further training sort of resents "another one of those." But I did know that if there was an ovarian cancer, it could potentially metastasize to the bone (the lumbar spine, for example) and cause low back pain. This young lady had been my patient for sometime (two to three years). If she had this, I might have been at fault for having not caught it earlier [about like the fellow with the testicular mass could honestly blame the doctors who missed it]. More importantly, she would surely suffer more because of my not becoming aware sooner.

In my examining her back, *she* asked permission to remove her bulky sweatshirt and did so. That left her with just her bra on, with the paper sheet covering her lower parts. About then, she (focused on back issues) also volunteered that someone had told her she might have scoliosis. On this I actually knew how to proceed. [That always brings comfort.] My friend and study group colleague, Genevieve, had taught our study group how to screen for scoliosis in medical school, and I had done this many times since. At the Europa clinic, we'd had a physiotherapist occupying an office within our clinic. His name was Steve, and I came to love and respect him. He married that other senior partner of mine, and they had a family. That proximity had allowed fairly quick consultations in this area, and I started to build my confidence in back exam, but I still wasn't adept.

So this patient hopped off the table [*and she may have set the sheet down*, though I couldn't later recall it – I was too focused on her medical problems], and I screened her for scoliosis by having her bend down toward touching her toes: her rib cage did not rise higher on one side than the other as one would see in an uncompensated scoliosis. So I resumed doing what I was able to by way of assessment of the back after she lay back down on her tummy with the sheet securely back on at that point when she announced that *she also had tender breasts*. Double poop! That meant a fifth symptom: constipation, left lower abdominal pain now with an ovarian mass (possibly causal), right lower back pain, possible scoliosis, and now breast tenderness. I felt some sense of being overwhelmed. [Move over resident physicians to Dr. House!] The uterus had not been enlarged on pelvic exam, but the left adnexal (fallopian tube or ovarian) mass might theoretically be an ectopic pregnancy. And *I had not had my staff do a pregnancy test* on her before they left – only a urinalysis. My oversight! She turned over and opened her bra so that I could do a breast exam. She did not have clinical signs of the breast changes consistent with pregnancy. She later said in court that I went on to fully remove her bra – that would CERTAINLY not be my nature. If the said bra had kept getting in the way of my exam and she wanted to help me, *I may have assisted her* in its removal. Not otherwise. I have no recall whether that was the case, in this instance. Don't you wish you had perfect detailed recall of everything that really turned out to matter later on, even if you didn't know it at the time?

She also said later in court that for a short time I palpated both her breasts at the same time. I have indeed done this occasionally to enable comparison of nodularities [breast lumpiness of the two sides should be in mirror images of each other] – so I may have done that this time. She said further that for a time when I did this my eyes were closed. And yes, I have done that also to avoid distraction during palpation, so I may have done that also on this occasion. *Do I recall* doing that in this instance? No. I don't really recollect much of the exam (much as I'd have liked to recall it).

I don't try to remember exams; patients don't want me to because then when I see them at the grocery store or at church they might get embarrassed. Indeed, I write down the positive findings then and there (not days later with a bottle of wine), and then I "fogetta bout it" (to quote Hugh Grant in his movie *Mickey Blue Eyes*). I still think people don't really want doctors to remember all their examination details. It is just physical and maybe only temporary. A person is more than the outward body. Certainly what is inward is so much more important. Too often we envy or condemn the outward. If we could only see that pleasant outward physical characteristics can harbor inward unfaithfulness, inconstancy, whininess, horrific envy, unwillingness to contribute, simple dumbness, a complaining attitude, the nationally renowned Alberta sense of "entitlement" . . . or even emptiness. Ask yourself, "What is underneath what we envy or condemn?"

So I cannot recall her. In any case, I did have two conclusions right then: (1) There could be very serious pathology in the left adnexa (the left fallopian tube and ovary), and (2) she must be worried [because I was]. I didn't have all of the answers, but I tried to reassure her by bending forward and softly speaking something consoling. Here, she (in court) describes things differently. She says that at this point, I lifted her off the table and began kissing her neck . . . soundlessly. Now *that's a fantasy!* Woe, where did it come from?! Were we both in the same reality dimension? *No, I didn't do that!* And I don't have to recall the actual exam to state that. I am really sure I would have remembered *that* little episode: it just did not happen! DC, that was, actually, something I was not physically able to do, but of course, you could not possibly know what my kisses sounded like. You have never received or heard one. My wife, and each of my children, knows what my kisses sound like. You don't!

In 1985, while I was a surgical resident at Dalhousie, I assisted Dr. Leo Bilodeau with perhaps six maxillofacial surgeries at the military hospital. Knowing he was good at the procedure, I consulted him in that regard for myself. I had an unyielding cross-bite that was causing progressive gum recession. He proposed that we do that surgery on me and also a wisdom tooth removal. He did a five-piece LeFort I procedure and a mandibuloplasty and dealt with the wisdom tooth in surgery in the summer of 1986. But with me there was a complication (of course); in cutting the maxilla into five parallel slices, *he made a hole in my hard palate*. In doing damage control, he put a type of crazy glue in the two centimeters acquired cleft palate he had made and provided an appliance to cover the hole. But I had to remove the appliance to enjoy meals. In the weeks after my start at Europa Medical Centre in Edmonton a few months later, my senior partner began teasing me about soup or carbonated beverage coming out of my right nostril during a meal (when I wouldn't use my appliance). It was so embarrassing! And I would never suck on a straw. After a couple of years, scar filled in all but a narrow passageway even though I had asked an ENT to attempt to close it surgically for me in 1988 – the attempt failed. But all I was left with in 1989 was a very narrow passageway between the roof of my mouth and my left maxillary sinus and nose. It caused a squeaky whistle when I kissed, cleared my palate, or drank with a straw. [And I've still got it now.] But I didn't make it public knowledge – it was embarrassing! And that complainant could never have known that what she accused me of was *impossible* for me. In fact, it didn't occur to me that this might be a factor in my defense. It was in the middle of a sleep one night that it occurred to me to ask my lawyer to inquire of her in the preliminary hearing what my kisses sounded like. I was so relieved to hear her commit herself, under oath, that *the kisses* she complained of *were silent*. It was on record.

As I had explained, my lawyer says that he felt this patient attended for more than medical care. As I said, he told me that out in my waiting room she had been reading a "romance novel." I don't know, but I was so grateful for that fine lawyer. I had never had lawyer experience except as social acquaintances and in buying a home. I have learned since knowing Bob White [I've got to provide his honorable name as well] that there are lawyers and there are LAWYERS. So I have thought about what he said many times. I have reflected and rereflected on this experience, which I could never unfortunately actually recall. Was the fantasy of flirting easier than the reality of a mass? Is it possible that she had understood that I was rejecting an advance on her part? *Did she feel jilted?* A more modern way of saying that is, did she feel dis'd – as in discarded or dismissed? I think of the phrase by William Congreve modified to, "Hell hath no fury as a woman scorned!" Did I do something in my prior contacts with her to permit her to believe that this married man was available for a romantic interest? If so, I would apologize from the depths of my soul to her . . . and [much more importantly] *to my wife*! You know what? I'm never going to know! I would like to talk with her about it someday . . . briefly . . . in a <u>very</u> public place. Perhaps even that would be unsafe for me.

In any case, I did not know which final diagnoses would be accurate. I held tight to the fact that there was a mass in the left adnexa (tube or ovary). There WAS pathology. I had unanswered questions, and *I was responsible for helping her.* A pelvic ultrasound would show a cystic or solid mass or an ectopic pregnancy. I hoped to arrange it the next day, but still . . . I expected some emotion from the patient – had she understood what I had told her? Why was there no emotion? Or had there been, and I don't recall? Was the possibility of a bad mass in her pelvis so fearful that she could not even *consider* it? Was there emotion that I did not see? Did she need to focus on the more "hopelessly" romantic theme: "I am so gorgeous that the doctor just had to hit on me" story? Had I used up all my usefulness to her by not being seduced? She certainly could have claimed that I had raped or tried to rape her. I had done a vaginal exam on her. Why the kissing thing? And only recently it has occurred to me – she may have figured that a raped label might make *her* less desirable to others while a stolen kiss – more desirable?

I did hear her girlfriend gush something akin to "Wow, can you imagine! Like, nothing like that ever happens to me!" later on the witness stand, in court. This was the girlfriend that she saw at West Edmonton Mall right after our appointment. But then, I think she told the story to several others. And I suspect those others didn't gush.

I wrote my notes and plans, and we left that Wednesday night with the plan that I would contact her the next day with an ultrasound appointment. She later said that I stayed in the room while she dressed, but *I would say* that IF that happened, it was she who chose to dress while I briefly wrote my notes (and I really wanted to get some notes down!). It's just a different point of view. The next day I called for an ultrasound. I really pressed that office for an urgent one and got it for the day following (a Friday). I had fully planned to go down the hall and observe the ultrasound while it was being done as I occasionally did when I was concerned so that I would have the results immediately and then bring the patient down the hall to formulate our plan. However, I just became too busy. The department did call the next afternoon with the confirmation that there were two large cysts on the left ovary: the larger being about five centimetres in diameter. That was felt to be a critical size in those days. No ectopic pregnancy, no solid tumor, just two cysts – one of which had gotten to critical size. And I trusted her. She said she was in pain and unable to work. I believed her. I had no reason not to.

So what can happen to a large cyst? It can twist on its blood supply (torsion), suddenly empty some or all of its contents (rupture), or undergo a bleed into its wall (become hemorrhagic). I asked a favor of one of my gynecology colleagues to see her urgently, but it would be after the weekend. Until she was seen by a specialist, *she was my responsibility.* I conscientiously did call the young woman with the appointment and to offer medication to get her through the weekend, but she declined this latter. Thankfully, when she was seen by my colleague, I had already completed the necessary investigations, so after also examining her, Dr. Mah simply put her on oral contraceptives to suppress the hormonal stimulus to form or grow cysts; despite the size of the cysts, no need for surgery. No need to drain the cysts. Excellent! I was content. I very much appreciated Dr. May-Sue Mah's kind assistance and asked this patient after, by phone, if she felt better now. She said she did. I asked myself the question, what complaint would there have been if she had had a solid mass with an associated cystic portion?

ACCUSED AND CHARGED PUBLICLY

However, I next heard about this patient through the Edmonton City Police, who charged me with sexual assault and arrested me. I was in the news: a scandal! Along with this scandalous report, the police, through their spokesman [whom I now know to have been Randy Kilburn], plead with the public to come forward if they had any "similar complaint" against me. In point of fact, Mr. Randy Kilburn later became my patient. This media appeal was very successful: another five of my patients complained about me. One had lost her first pregnancy and blamed me for it. One had apparently felt aroused as I explained and demonstrated her sexual dysfunction to her with her husband by my side. An older woman said she felt *I had been rough* physically as I examined her with palpation and had recalled my review of lab work with her but felt that I had said your vaginal orgasms are normal rather than "your vaginal organisms [flora] are normal." A woman at the Misericordia Hospital Staff Health Office complained that she had had the required pelvic exam, even though she was still menstruating a bit. I had carefully reviewed the form that required completion for employment. Yes, a pelvic exam [but no speculum exam, Pap smear, or swab] needed to be done before she could be employed, and she had said she couldn't come back after her period was over. For me blood is not an issue, but I realize that I am not as "grossed out" by it as the lay public might be. A friend of the lady, who had accused me of kissing her, also lodged a complaint – that my pelvic exam for her presenting complaint of vaginal pain with the onset of intercourse was *so gentle* it reminded her of lovemaking. Oh my goodness; for some I was too rough and for others too gentle. One lady complained that she had been assaulted by hundreds of physicians, and now she complained of me too. Remember the cascade or domino effect. It had happened again to me because the media frenzy made Edmonton a small town. The media had all the answers! The WHOLE story! I think you get the picture. Another patient went to the media and got her story in the paper first *before* going to the police. And further, one saw an opportunity to make some money that she really needed, and her despair made her willing to concoct a zinger of a tale. The media loved the stories from these nine eventual accusers.

But I was terrified. I knew that I would need legal help, but with such a throng of accusers, who would want to take the case? Clarence Darrow is credited with saying, "Lost causes are the only ones worth fighting for." An acquaintance/friend who was a lawyer asked if I would like him to defend me. I didn't really know anything about his legal skills, but I had faith in him, as a person. He, actually, was great at his job but probably knew that our "friendship" would fade as he did what had to be done to defend me. Still he realized that I needed someone gifted in the law more than a friend, and without false humility, he knew that he was good. He tried to enable me to stay away from the media – taking taxis from loading docks at the law courts building, for example, to avoid the prying eyes and exploitive cameras. The questions! His rule was that I speak with no one about my side of the accusations. There were dozens of calls to my office from the media. They wanted my side of the story, but I declined to provide comment or even talk with them, as my lawyer advised. He needed to control information from me. It was scary for Dianne and I to plan to avoid the paparazzi of our city. They didn't want calmly conveyed information; they wanted something to print or televise. They twice set up a television camera in the hall outside the door of my office and began filming and questioning the people who were coming in. Stan, the pharmacist downstairs, an owner of the building and friend came up and told them to leave the building. He was quite firm. I wondered if some vigilante might try to harm me for what the media had conveyed my character to be. I wanted to hide. I wanted to stay in bed or under it. Well, I couldn't do that because we had a waterbed.

The media loved its position of high moral ground. It could feign alarm and horror about sexual exploitation by a doctor on pages 1-5, and then they could advertise sexually explicit movies and escort services or exotic dance clubs deeper in the pages of the paper and charge more due to their expanded readership. It was good for business. Sex sells. On TV, some media correspondent would voice the public's outrage on the six or eleven o'clock news, and then that same channel would be advertising telephone sex just a few hours later. I wonder if they ever recognized this obvious behavioral inconsistency. In what ways is being falsely accused of sexual assault, like being sexually assaulted?

My then ten-year-old son Michael had a paper route. I usually helped him deliver his papers. How heart wrenching for both of us when his dad's picture was on the front page of the two city papers with the horrible accusations – not just of unfaithfulness to his mother [I feel sympathy for the *children* of Tiger Woods] but aggression against women at large. He suggested we cut out these articles from each paper before we delivered his papers. I loved him the more for his brave protective instinct, but we didn't do the snipping thing. We just *trudged* out there to get the paper out to our neighbors. Those were hard times for Dianne, me, and the children. We were under attack but couldn't provide ourselves strength in numbers by hanging out together all the time. I had to keep going to work to maintain some status quo. Dianne had to stay at home to maintain its environment. The children had to go to school. We tried to avoid the media because whenever they caught a glimpse of us, we would be on the news again that night. One day as I went into work from the parking lot, a furtive figure arose from between vehicles. I did not recognize the bearded face, but felt sure that someone had risen to the task of meting out social justice to the "doctor who did foul things to women." He began to raise from an area hidden from my view, what I figured must be a shotgun. In that second, I thought I was going to die. I decided that if I was to die, it would be with a greeting on my lips. So I called out a hearty hello to him and walked straight toward him as he raised his . . . news camera. I continued as I had begun and extended my hand to him and said a loud "Good morning!" That clip never was shown on TV. It was probably "not evil enough." But other pictures with their condemning narratives did make the news. So we learned to keep *TRUDGING* along.

THE RULE OF THIRDS AND THE FIRST TRIAL

My children had to face the children of people who read or watched the news. Those parents/people formed opinions. Everyone forms opinions. This is Canada! I was news. Even some "friends" at church distanced themselves from me. They were, after all, church people. What I had been accused of was against the *tenets of our faith*. Small wonder some of them felt uncomfortable or unsafe around me. *It wasn't very Christian of them to shun me, BUT it was very human!* Some doctors also shunned me. To many, I was a pariah, a leper. Remember, I had wanted to end my relationship with that senior partner of mine after he had had "impossible to consent to" sexual relations with his patient in his at-home additional office. Small wonder that some in the medical community wanted to ostracize me. They didn't know much about me and feared what they did not know. More recently, I was told by the leaders of an Edmonton-area physicians network: "*You* would not be welcome." No room for explanation or evidence. That was hardly important to them. I was painfully taught the rule of thirds: when someone is accused of wrong, one-third of his prior acquaintances will condemn, one-third will defend, and one-third will pick his conversations for little morsels of gossip [probably the most painful] to spread about; and those who comprise each third will not be predictable based on past interactions. But then, what about those who had never even known me before? *They just assumed* that with the media junk, *they did KNOW* me!

It took about three years to get through the criminal court system and be given a "directed verdict"! That meant that we didn't even have to present a legal defense. The prosecution's case "didn't hold water," to quote from the movie *My Cousin Vinny*. That year, Dianne and I had Keltie, our ninth child, because we were still devoted to and in love with each other. And we felt that our main purpose in life is to become good parents, as we are parented from above. Our children continued to be a consequence of our love. I worry that my anxieties and stress may have made me (or Dianne) less available to them, though. That saddens me, even now. Then it was another year 'til the Supreme Court said that a directed verdict could not be done, in this instance. Before we received that crushing news, however, the college had its disciplinary hearing over these same accusations because *they wanted to be seen to be doing* something. Only two of the nine witnesses were willing to testify at the college hearing because there was no longer a media frenzy about me: only the girl whose report had started the cascade and her friend [chapter 5, reason 2]. The college was really not supposed to proceed until the criminal proceedings were over, but they were anxious to please the political public. They heard for the first time that I could not do what I had been accused of. But this occurred, only at the cost of my further loss of privacy. The cat was out of the bag; our "secret" was told to the college and from the college to the ear of the criminal prosecutor. We could never again surprise the prosecution with that fact.

The college, in its turn, eventually judged that I had *not been sufficiently sensitive* to the modesty of my patients with adequate draping, that my manner had allowed my patients to feel caressed, and that I "had *remained in the room*" to write my notes and discuss plans while a patient dressed. By doing this, they could show to the public due diligence by suspending me for six months, and then set aside that suspension if I would

1. be assessed by a world class psychiatric institution for detection of predatory personality traits and
2. have my clinical practice skills assessed by medical evaluators.

I did this, and they both said I was OK, but for my OCD traits (my obsessiveness). So I continued to practice as before, except for my abiding some private legal advice from my lawyer, Mr. Bob White, with regard to things to avoid.

THE SECOND TRIAL

Then, the Supreme Court made its determination, and so we had another three years of court preparation, motions, and a second trial – this time including all the young military girls from years before, who sat just outside the court room and chatted together as a group before giving their evidence. I guess it was no big surprise that *this time when they were witnesses, they all said the same thing*: that in my interactions with them those many years before, I had had (in each and every instance) a penile erection that they saw or that I rubbed on them. New heights of embarrassment! The same story came from each one. Do they have any idea how impossibly demanding a "constant state of arousal" would have been to any living man – well . . . over age fourteen? Moreover, that had specifically been denied during the investigation by the military police. I suppose the embellishment was what they felt was their *civic duty* [chapter 5, reason 2] in the putting away of a "dangerous criminal" – me! I didn't feel dangerous. I didn't even scare myself. Despite surviving the pain of previously hurt feelings, it was painful to hear. Again! And again the media had a heyday! Dianne, I, and the children went through several more weeks of stress and grief. The impossibility of having done that of which I had been accused was no surprise this time but still incontrovertible. Still, there was the inevitable strain before being found *not guilty of any of the charges*, finally in 1996. We won our case. I could stand tall . . . but I felt short and bent. I was worn-out. I really needed a break. I had kept up my practice, including obstetrics, through it all. I was exhausted. To celebrate and relax, I took my wife and children to Disneyland, Universal Studios, and Knott's Berry Farm. We loved that trip together! By then, our Becky was nineteen, Michael was seventeen, Amy was almost sixteen, Leisl was fourteen, Shawn was twelve, David was ten, Cameron was eight, Marcus was seven, and Keltie was four years old. The worth of these children was so much greater than the world's favor. Each of the children had their assigned buddies, and Dianne and I had the youngest two. It was a restorative trip for the family. In Disneyland no one had seen pictures or heard stories about me. They had other things to be ecxited about. I was just another dad/husband with a bunch of kids.

POSTTRIAL LIFE WITHIN THE CLOUD OF ACCUSATION

However, as I have previously said, many persons with no direct knowledge of any of the facts had chosen sides – several doctors and nurses among them. They had judiciously or maliciously presided over their own "trials by media" and "trials by hearsay." Medical people like to be right even relying on the sordid media or covert reports from a friend of a friend or "what some patient told a friend of mine." Oh, the media! The media! They knew that scandalous reporting increased readership or viewing. They knew that I would be *unable to provide* any countering evidence while criminal proceedings were in process. And *that was fine* by them. They could print the outlandish, the fantastic, and the sensational, and then say or write that I had been unwilling or unavailable to comment [say anything to the contrary] in defense. So I must have been guilty, right? 'Cause "where there's smoke, there's fire," right? [Don't you just love little proverbs? They can easily replace a lack of any truth.]

Armed with those proverbs and media "evidence," we don't really need due process, facts, or assumptions of innocence. *Everyone, who is ever accused, must be guilty.* Just hang 'em here and now. In fact, the registrar of the College of Physicians and Surgeons of Ontario had been quoted as saying generally that if a woman ever made a sexual complaint, he knew "in his heart of hearts" that it was true. No need for evidence, hearings, or due process. It was a time of social change. Glen Gabbard wrote and was quoted extensively on sexual exploitation by an authority figure. I purchased and read one of his books to understand the social trend and the nature of the accusation against me. The idea of zero tolerance emerged. Organizations for the protection of women, particularly, were upset – not because they knew specific facts, but because I was a focus of the sociopolitical issue. I had been accused, and my accusers should be believed, no matter what they said.

I was personally *convinced that many women had been abused* by those in authority, caregivers, and some occasional physicians (see my notes about my previous senior partner). The college actually came up with a very sensitizing poster of a young waif in distress that read, "I was a patient of Dr. XXX, until . . ." They wanted this poster hung in every office in the province. That pretty well identified a vulnerable point for all male doctors thereafter. I wondered if I was to be sacrificed on the altar of social conscience and change – simply for being there at that time.

However, the "sides" had been chosen, and medical people don't often back down. In contrast, a young doctor across the hall, Dr. Fraser Armstrong [whom I am proud to name], had refused to accept any patients who wanted to leave my care. This man had honor! In the end, thirty-four people from my practice did change physicians. The vast majority *continued to believe in me.* God bless them for their loyalty. Some others not in my practice, including doctors and nurses, believed the media – and this is the time that evidence-based medicine had begun to become important. But a need for evidence didn't influence *those* groups of nurses or physicians. Evidence was just needed for medicine in their minds, not for juicy community gossip. This also applied to some parents at the schools of our children and some lawyers 'cause they had received their "evidence" from a "usually reliable source" (the media) after all. My family was told that people would gradually forget. And perhaps they did, over time. But what the public might have eventually forgotten, the lawyers didn't forget. "I could have convicted him," some thought. I think many envied the skills of Mr. Bob White as well they might. He was very good at his job. I am sure he could have convicted me or defended me from conviction, such was his skill.

CHANGES MADE

I went back to working after the Disneyland trip. The years rolled by. What had I learned, even right from the start of those early accusations, in 1989? Here is a short list:

1. *Always use a chaperone* even if a senior partner tells you not to – in the hospital, in the office, if you are called in, or doing a home visit. I installed phone jacks in all my exam rooms so that my staff/chaperones could be in the rooms with me for any woman in a state of undress or exposure. My wife and daughters, in addition to my other paid staff, all became chaperones for me.
2. Keep most patients wearing as much of their own clothing as possible. *Never let them inadequately drape themselves* again! Don't expose them unnecessarily – even to the chaperone. Push clothing out of the way, with permission, rather than remove it.
3. Good people might be willing to embellish their story, if they really believed that they can *help someone else achieve justice who actually might* have been harmed [chapter 5, reason 2]. Then, if they lie, they are really not liars – just noble helpers!
4. Most people are good and basically honest. But the good ones don't always wear a label. So be careful.
5. *Always ask permission* to lift a shirt or skirt or undo a bra – even with the chaperone present.
6. Some patients might make a claim simply for litigation purposes. They have borrowed from the trend in the USA.
7. I hadn't really *learned much about back assessment* from medical training up to 1989.

So these were my realizations. *What did I do about it?*

1. I determined to always use a chaperone unless declined. And I have, except one glaring time when I thought it was being declined (about which I will tell you later).

2. As much as possible, I kept patients dressed, just *undoing or pushing aside* what they agreed to for the purpose of the exam.

3. And I sought to learn more: specifically, *more training in back assessment*. This I secured by doing CME. That means continuing medical education. The truth is that I tried to do the CME in Edmonton, among those whom I thought were my colleagues, but it often made me uncomfortable. Perhaps, I became paranoid about the whisperings of some of the other doctors. I found it was distracting. Everywhere, except at the family practice rounds at the Alex. The doctors at the Alex seemed to continue to accept me as a colleague. Some joked with me in the hallways. They would work alongside me. They would train alongside me. They were friendly and supportive in the meetings. But I needed CME outside the Alex, and meetings arranged by the College of Family Physicians of Canada were so often very uncomfortable: it was hard to learn because of the unfriendliness and clear condemnatory attitudes of some "now indignant because they had not been right" Edmonton physicians who also attended these conferences. Dr. Doug Armstrong – not from my hospital – was a remarkable exception, as also his son, Fraser. So were Ken Gardiner, Dave Adams, and Doug Perry. What remarkable men! *They didn't seem convinced by the media.* They believed in the law and that one was innocent until proven guilty. I had pondered: am I not human? "Hath not an accused, eyes? Hath not an accused, hands, organs, dimensions, senses, affections, passions? Fed with the same food, hurt with the same weapons, subject to the same means, warmed and cooled by the same winter and summer, as an unaccused? If you prick us, do we not bleed?" (corrupted from William Shakespeare's *Merchant of Venice*). I guess those "few good men" really made *evidence-based* decisions. That was refreshing. *But I did need more education.* I needed to keep updating. I needed knowledge. For those who continued to believe in me, I had to be current. *I needed to learn how to do a proper diagnostically organized back exam.* I had to go outside Edmonton, outside Alberta, even outside Canada.

KEEPING CURRENT

I attended pediatrics, obstetrics and gynecology conferences in Regina or Saskatoon (abbreviated POGO). I attended internal medicine updates for those preparing for their fellowship exams presented by the University of Utah. I went to conferences at the Mayo Clinic. I went to the American Academy of Family Physicians (AAFP) Annual Scientific Assemblies in various sites that were affordable. Dianne always went with me and did some of the offered tours and courses. Those were our only outings together without the children. How I looked forward to having time with her. At those American Academy courses, there were *excellent lectures and updates*. Many original researchers gave lectures or talks. There were tens of thousands of physicians in the AAFP organization, so they could "afford" world-renowned experts. I smile, even now, when I think of the excellence of that type of teaching/training.

About one-third of the AAFP membership were DOs [DOs are Doctors of Osteopathy], and the other two-thirds were MDs. Early in my attendance in these courses, I noticed a considerable amount of musculoskeletal training, and that included back examinations and treatments. Just what I needed to learn more about. I attended courses in issues regarding the cervical spine, the thoracic spine, the lumbar spine, and the sacroiliac joints. I was taught *spray and stretch* technique. I began to be taught that fibrous ligamentous tissue could actually be specifically enhanced or redeposited where previous trauma had damaged it. The process was called prolotherapy and offered new nonsurgical therapy to patients with excessively mobile joints. In the end, I truly became one of those "MEN IN B[L]ACK." [Sorry for that – I tell my kids that's "Dad humor."]

CHAPTER 3

WHAT WAS THEN, THAT ONE TIME THAT I DIDN'T USE A NEEDED CHAPERONE, AFTER 1996?

I DID GET LOTS of training in back exams. I learned of and developed an *interest in manual therapy*, which could help people in pain without drugs. My training for this came through CME, largely enabled by the American Academy of Family Physicians, of whom a third of the members were osteopaths. As I studied with them, I was not seen as a pariah. I had *painfully* had my picture in the papers and my face on television in trial. Nonetheless, at AAFP, *I allowed* that my picture be taken learning manual therapy for back dysfunction and used in the syllabus the following year for advertisement. I completed several courses in that interest area, the more recent ones being taught by doctors of osteopathy. The techniques that I acquired did not have their origins in one single discipline. So I am a hybrid (or a mongrel)! I had learned from physiotherapists, physiatrists, orthopedic medicine (Cyriax) physicians, prolotherapists, and doctors of osteopathy. I have learned that Western and Eastern Europe have many contributions to make in terms of herbal medicine awareness and manual medicine.

It just didn't make sense anymore to think of medicine being owned regionally. It didn't make sense to sneer at others trained elsewhere because they didn't use the same textbook I used. Who knows, maybe the text they trained from was better.

Although I had begun timorously from 1991, I used manual medicine more and more in my practice. By January 2000, I was finding manual therapy very satisfying and a strong asset to my family practice. I was, however, aware that some of my local colleagues might not even feel comfortable reducing dislocated shoulders or elbows, so I had to be sure that I never did harm because if harm is apparently caused, then the uninformed have fuel for their criticism. Consider for a moment the huge rift that was allowed to grow up between traditional medicine and chiropractic practice in Canada. Some taught that those "lesser practitioners" were to be distained [rather like the Catholics and the protestants in Ireland – an *Us versus Them* game]. On the other hand, I have no real idea what percentage of physicians in Edmonton do manual medicine for their patients. In any case, I now had to practice flawlessly. I had no room for any mistakes because I had previously been so scrutinized. I still made a mistake.

THE GOOD SAMARITAN

On Friday, 21 January '00, I was working at one of the two hospitals at which I had privileges: the Royal Alexandra in Edmonton. I was writing notes in a patient's chart on a side counter. A nurse whom I did not know was also making notes in a chart, seated at the unit desk. Although she noted that she had visibly taken medication in her complaint letter, I did not see that, and that was not what drew my attention to her. She gained my notice by reaching behind herself, rubbing her upper back, twisting her back and chest thrusting in an obviously distressed fashion.

I left open the chart that I had been writing in and went to her side. I identified myself (I was also wearing my white lab coat and photo ID) and asked if she was all right. She informed me that she wasn't and explained that she had back pain. To my further inquiry, she explained that the site of the back pain was between her shoulder blades. I knew that many of those kinds of problems could easily be resolved by manual therapy.

I explained to her that I do some training in manual medicine and osteopathy, and that I might be able to help her. She accepted my offer to help, so I looked for a nearby place where brief privacy could be afforded. The obvious site was a few steps away in what looked like the supply room. In her letter of complaint, she referred to it as the printer room. Maybe it was both. I saw that it was well lit and empty. I pulled the blinds closed to ensure privacy, closed the door, and asked her to undo her uniform so I could see her back. She consented and did so. Just as I started to ask, "Is there someone you'd like to stand in as a chaperone?" she exclaimed that she would "just die if someone walked in."

I took that as a request for privacy, *and also to mean that she didn't want to involve a chaperone*, although she did not specifically state that. She describes this in a slightly different way in her letter of complaint: "I said I didn't want anyone coming in and getting the wrong idea because my shirt was undone, and he said fine and put his back to the door."

I replied in writing that "I therefore put my foot against the door to ensure we would not be interrupted. I requested that she come to where I was standing and face away from me." With her permission, I lifted the back of her front-unbuttoned uniform top. I asked if I could open the clasp of her bra to uncover her back, to which she verbally agreed.

COLLEGE AND REGION EXAMINE MY TECHNIQUE (2000)

Now I am going to quote from my exact written response to the college as I describe what they would *then* have known about my technique *as of my letter March 5, 2000*: "I do the assessment for this problem by putting my left hand on the *skin* overlying the low sternum and with my right hand palpate beside the Spinous Processes of the thorax with the index and long finger tips. I simply feel for asymmetry in (tissue) muscle tone one site at a time until I have palpated paraspinously the entire thoracic spine: it would take 10–15 seconds.

I am checking for *the level* at which I first encounter (from the bottom upwards) increased paraspinous muscle tone and *the side* that I note it on. I also have a clinical impression (by the chest hand) whether there is any costochondritis or rib subluxation [plus the presence of rib fracture or deformity, but I didn't write that at the time]. It has been my experience that doing a 'thrust maneuver', with either [and, in retrospect, any of the three] of these present will actually *increase* the pain and contribute to inflammation.

If the (tissue) tone is increased at, say, a T7 or T8 site, I would proceed differently than for a T3 or T4 site. Although because of the sheer number of times I have done this therapy I do not remember the precise level or side in this specific instance, I can describe what would have happened. I would have asked that she place the hand of the affected side on the opposite shoulder, and the other hand (then) on the opposite shoulder. Then (and this, of course, takes her complete cooperation), I would reach around from behind her and draw the elbows toward their opposite sides (with my hands) and with the front of my chest to her back, do the thrust maneuver."

OK. That's it. That is what I had provided the college in terms of my technique. That is what they knew for sure: my *exactly described technique*. And I easily acknowledge that in the doing of this, my left hand has to make some contact with the breast margins often. Do you understand that they knew exactly my approach to the problem? This was in the year 2000. Now, in response to my written explanation, the assistant registrar met with me and asked me to demonstrate the technique on him. I asked him to please *unbutton his shirt*, which he declined to do – he said words to the effect: "The college has no problem with skin-to-skin contact, but I'm not going to have you do it that way on me. Just proceed as you would if I had." So I put my left hand on his low sternum and the sites of chondrosternal joining and with my right hand tried to palpate through his shirt(s), differences in paraspinous tissue tone [although I wasn't experienced at through-clothing palpation]. And you know what? I felt one! He had a somatic dysfunction of the thoracic spine! I don't recall the level or the side, but he had one. So I was able to walk him through the way I would proceed and actually manipulate his back resulting in an improvement, which he acknowledged. He repeated that the college had no problem with my use of skin-to-skin contact. He told me that he thought I had explained well how I was going to proceed. He called this a "running commentary" and advised me to continue to do that with patients. However, because of the fact that this contact was made with a staff person at the RAH, the hospital administration had also launched their own investigation. They, also, got basically the same information from the two of us.

In her letter of complaint, her last paragraph says that she "was shocked that he had put his hands [although in the early text she acknowledges that it was just one hand] on my chest and embarrassed. I have been seeing chiropractors and massage therapists for years and have never felt uncomfortable or embarrassed. I spoke with my chiropractor, Dr XXXX who said there was no reason that he could think of for not adjusting my back through my clothes, there is no reason for undoing my shirt or bra."

I have actually attended lectures by chiropractors, and one of them said he does no assessment whatsoever before beginning some manipulations. Fascinating, but that is not what I had been taught. So what is this about? I had done it differently than she was used to. My approach was much more cautious than that with which she was familiar. And a trusted chiropractor, rather than diffusing the situation by telling her, "Well, there certainly are a lot of ways to do assessments and manual therapy," said instead something that made her feel badly about me and badly about herself having allowed me to proceed that way. I suggest that it is this type of professional commentary that contributes to, and may even *produce*, hurt and complaints. Where there might initially have been questions, there was hurt after. I suggest that my "Good Samaritan" offer was made and carried out with only good intent. I suggest that my assessment made only one manipulation necessary and that my service did overcome her back problem. And she does agree with this. I suggest that this was offered in the spirit of collegiality. I suggest that if her chiropractor had proceeded in a more flexible way, the concern would have stopped there. Why did he not? There are at least two reasons:

1. He felt that manual therapy was his turf and wanted to protect it (and hence, his income).
2. He may have only been aware of his discipline's approach to that clinical problem and perhaps has never been informed of other techniques and methods.

Can you think of other explanations?

COLLEGE AND REGION CONFIRM TECHNIQUE

Well, in the end, I received two letters: the first, from Dr. XXXX for the hospital administration and, the second, from Dr. YYYY for the college. You now know that they were each aware of my exact technique. Here quoted are their concluding letters to me, dated 28 March 2000 and 15 May 2000, respectively.

> From XXXX, MD
> Executive Vice-President, Chief Clinical Officer – Capital Health and Associate Dean, Clinical Affairs, Faculty of Medicine and Dentistry – University of Alberta
>
> Dear Dr. Litchfield
>
> I have reviewed the information provided to me as a result of the investigation into the complaint received alleging inappropriate behaviour by you towards an employee of the Royal Alexandra Hospital.
>
> I have determined that the particular method of osteopathy treatment that you provided to the employee *does not appear to be out of line in terms of normal practice*. However, I would recommend the following guidelines to you in order to prevent similar complaints in the future:

- In all cases, it is *advisable to at least offer*, if not insist, that *another female be present whenever treatment involving skin to skin contact* is administered to females. It is recommended that you consider this even when offering treatment to the staff in your practice.
- As a matter of course, it is recommended that you provide thorough and consistent explanation [Author's Note: this is kind of like the 'running commentary' theme] of the treatment you are about to administer, and to obtain express consent from the recipient. It is not advisable to assume that the recipient may have more understanding of the process because of their involvement or familiarity with medical services. In this particular circumstance, the individual had previously received treatment in a different way than administered by you, and explanation may have prevented surprise and questions when the treatment differed from the individual's previous experience.
- There is the potential of liability and/or dissatisfaction with outcome whenever offering treatment, even if this is done as a favour to an employee. Therefore, whenever medical services are provided to anyone, a consistent process should be followed which includes explanation to the recipient of the treatment, obtaining the recipient's consent to the proposed treatment, and documenting a record of the treatment provided.
- I trust that you will incorporate these recommendations into your practice. I have now concluded my investigation, and you are free to assume treatment of any of your patients who are, or who become inpatients at the Royal Alexandra Hospital.

Yours sincerely,

So what is there here? An affirmation that *the "particular method of osteopathy that I used was not out of line,* in terms of normal practice." There is (1) a (again) guideline to use a *chaperone for any skin-to-skin contact* examination or treatment (which I had intended to do in this case); (2) a caution to never assume that they know anything, but explain carefully what you are going to do and obtain agreement/ consent for *TREATMENT*; and (3) a recommendation to document the encounter.

THERE IS NOT written (a) *a reproof for skin-to-skin contact* to the sternum or the back; (b) *a specific requirement for "consent for skin-to-skin contact"* which the committee will later maintain that there was; nor (c) *a criticism of my manual therapy technique.* You may need to go over the letter a couple of times to be sure that I have summarized it correctly. Go ahead, take your time. Next:

> From Dr YYYY, MB ChB
> Assistant Registrar
> College of Physicians and Surgeons
> Province of Alberta
>
> Dear Dr. Litchfield:
>
> I am writing in follow-up to our recent meeting to discuss the issues surrounding Ms ABCDs' complaint against you in respect of the care you provided to her.
>
> You indicated to me that it was your intention to help out a colleague who appeared to be in pain, and that you believed you had a skill set which could assist her in pain relief. You have acknowledged to me that your provision of these services fell below an accepted standard in that *the location* at which you provided the service was inappropriate, and that you had not *adequately clarified whether the patient wished for a chaperone* to be present.

You also indicated to me that you wish me to pass on your apologies to the complainant for any embarrassment which you may have caused her.

I must emphasize to you that, *recognizing your previous history with the College*, it is incumbent on you to ensure that chaperones are made available to all your female patients should they so wish. [And there it is: the formal administrative mention of my past publicly renowned media accusations!] There may be occasions, particularly in true emergency situations, where the accommodation of the patient's wish for a chaperone might not be reasonable and, your professional judgment would need to be used in such cases.

I would appreciate your providing me with your written confirmation that you will, in future, ensure that your female patients are offered a chaperone in any situation where there may be physical contact between you and the patient. This file will be closed upon receipt of your undertaking.

Sincerely,

And then, on May 23, 2000:

Thank you for your letter of May 17, 2000, received at this office on May 23, 2000. I appreciate your providing me with your undertaking. This file will now be closed.

Sincerely,

All right! First let me say that I thought Dr. YYYY had a very gentle personality, and he did engender an atmosphere of communication and trust, but he was not the BIG DOG, so he didn't make the final decisions. He took his information to the complaints' chairman. But what is in his direction? (1) A criticism for using the storage/computer room for this quick assessment (even if my foot against the door did ensure privacy). And I agree; it would have been much better if we had gone down to the emergency room briefly and (2) an insistence that I use a chaperone. Can you see anything else directed to me here?

WHAT THE REGION AND THE COLLEGE WANTED

So what is the <u>TOTAL DIRECTION</u> received from Dr. XXXX and from Dr. YYYY:

Dr. XXXX	Dr. YYYY
1. Insistence on chaperone to be present for treatment involving Skin-to-skin contact administered to female patients.	1. another female (chaperone)
2. Thorough and consistent explanation of treatment, with the obtaining of express consent.	
3. A documenting record	4. Use appropriate assessment locations.

Now *why is there a difference* aside from the documenting record and location appropriateness? Can you guess? Yes, of course, you can see it! Dr. XXXX talks about a thorough and consistent explanation of treatment with the obtaining of consent while Dr. YYYY does not. Why is that? They are certainly both bright doctors. Why the difference? I think I know.

Dr. YYYY had had the procedure done on himself (apart from the opening of his shirt, although he had said that the college did not have a problem with skin-to-skin contact), and he KNEW that *I automatically provide a running commentary and obtain consent* as I had done with him. He had congratulated me on my running commentary. It left nothing to the imagination. It was very concise. It is what I go through *with every patient new* to my brand of manual therapy. He could easily consent because I had explained it so well. This is necessary to all practitioners of manual medicine in order to get the patient cooperation necessary to do these interventions. Patients would never have any idea what position they needed to get into next, if there were no "running commentary." And if at any point a patient cries out, "Wait, wait! I'm not comfortable with this" (which some have done), then I don't proceed. Later in the findings of the committee, I was reprimanded for not providing *ANY* running commentary or explanation and not providing *ANY* informed consent.

- No running commentary – page 29 of the second transcript
- No running commentary – page 78 and on, of the second transcript
- No running commentary – page 150 of the second transcript

I had, unfortunately, pled guilty at my contracted lawyer's behest to not providing an *adequate* explanation for the need for a pelvic floor exam to the lady with piriformis syndrome. I realize now, however, that with the chatting of this patient she or the nurse present may simply not have heard, or registered, whatever I did say. I had, similarly, plead guilty to not going through an *adequate* informed consent with that same lady for the manual therapy. I did tell her about the need for me to "check the pelvic floor by doing a vaginal exam" and then did the manual therapies that might help her. Perhaps that was not "adequate" . . . perhaps. But I certainly did provide the running commentary FOR WHICH THE college had asked with opportunity for disconsent (which was probably not a word, until now). *Consent had, of course, been received* when she signed the back of the emergency registration form. At any time she could withdraw consent verbally, but she had given consent with her signature: "for any assessment or treatment that her attending physician deemed necessary."

The key here is "adequate"; I wasn't sure that the running commentary that the college and the Regional Health Authority had asked of me – and which I provided – was adequate. So I did agree to the guilty plea with the proviso that it read "adequate" rather than "no" explanation of consent. Furthermore, it had been the college who instructed me to use the running commentary. *And a written consent had been given.*

The lawyer for the college, of course, took it a step further and said that I had given *NO explanation* and went through *NO process of informed consent.* He also brought back Dr. XXXX and Dr. YYYY to ask them to rework their evidence and rethink "what they had meant" by their letters. I personally felt that their views five years later weren't the guidelines that I had been given, and you now have a copy of their original letters to me. Counsel for the college could not just allow that I had pled partially guilty to those charges. He had to make it sound much worse than I had admitted. He postulated that I had been *advised,* nay *commanded to provide* a "running commentary" to patients for manual therapy, and in his view, *I HAD NOT DONE SO!* There it is, counsel – you got me! I didn't do what I had been counseled strongly to do and then I just invaded the privacy of those women. It has the air of being convincing, doesn't it? I was told how to proceed, and my evil or unyielding nature stopped me. That's got to be it, doesn't it, counsel? Well, hang me high! I must be ever so guilty. I am pretty well agreeing with you . . . except . . . I do have just one question. I know that the nurse present didn't remember under oath all of my "running commentary" to our friend, the lady with piriformis syndrome, but might this have been because the lady kept chattering and distracting her? If she had remembered, then maybe the administration and the college would have had to "lose her" as a witness too. [It is possible that this is a little sarcastic.] But listen. *If I did not provide a running commentary, then how did that lady get into the right positions for manual therapy?* If I didn't explain that to check the pelvic floor, a vaginal exam was in order, then *why did she slip off her panties and prepare* for one? If I wasn't explaining step by step what we were going to do and how she should prepare herself, then how did she know what position to assume? Was it magic? Were the laws of (random positioning and) physics just suspended in that hospital right at that moment (this is also kind of borrowed from *My Cousin Vinny*)? If I didn't give an explanation and request to the woman who removed her panties and got into the lithotomy position for the pelvic exam, then something else must have prompted her, right then. What do you think, counsel? Maybe she was just coincidentally overly warm *right that minute* and wanted to cool down? To quote Tim Robbins in the *Shawshank Redemption* again: "How can you be so obtuse?" (And I guess that wasn't one question but seven, plus the one about your obtuseness.)

Now the blockbuster! As of May 15, 2000, the college and the region knew <u>fully</u> of my technique in this kind of back exam and said it was OK, yet proceeded with charging me for it for February 1, 2001 (nine months later), September 1, 2001 (sixteen months later), and December 30, 2001 (nineteen months later) with three counts of "on or about <u>month/day/year</u>, while examining your patient, (<u>various names)</u>, your method of examination did not conform with current medically accepted standards in that you did conduct an examination of your patient's back in such a manner that your hand contacted the bare breast of your patient."

That is *three allegations* of proceeding with back exams inappropriately *within nineteen months of their having carefully examined the technique and not having found anything wrong with it!* You read the advice they provided – I still have their original letters. About here, you must really be shaking your head. I know I was. What was this college about?

CHAPTER 4

WHAT'S THE COLLEGE ABOUT?

MY COLLEGE OF Physicians and Surgeons had, and still may have, in its entrance foyer a sign proclaiming its mandate: To "protect the public and *Provide Ethical Guidance* to the profession." Who could possibly argue with that dual mandate's appropriateness? It sounds exceptionally lofty . . . *and it is*. The college as an institution deserves our gratitude and respect. It is meant to keep order and appropriateness in the medical profession. That is why it must proceed very ethically in its affairs.

I have chosen to abide every order of the College, even though I have disagreed with them, because I believe in the organization (with one bylaw exception). And also really, I had no choice. I truly do like to be right. I'm sure my children never did notice that about me. And now as they grow and mature and start families, I believe I have noted an interest in being RIGHT among them. Nevertheless, although physicians like to be RIGHT, physicians are human – the humanness means that we are going to be wrong some of the time. Even the humans in the College of Physicians and Surgeons will be wrong some of the time. Imagine that! One always hopes that the entire Council of the College is not individually wrong all *at the same time*. But the Council of the College can be misled. An incorrect leader can have great sway. He can *make a wrong decision appear to be a cause célèbre*.

Colleges of physicians and surgeons are made up of two types of doctor. Those who are "permanent" (the registrar and his or her associates/assistants) and those who are elected for perhaps a couple of years – the "part-timers" (they form the Council of the College). Final decision-making power is *intended* to abide with the Council of the College: the elected part-timers! Nonetheless, due to experience, the permanent ones kind of provide training and direction to the part-timers – they "show them the ropes." Sometimes the training is formal, and sometimes the training is over coffee. When a registrar has coffee with you as you become a part-timer, you listen. He influences you. He may not say you must vote this way or that blatantly, but *he/she influences you*. Make no mistake!

Having all powers (executive, legislative, and judicial) would allow a person, for example, to propose a bylaw that every physician had to actively assist any pregnant patient to secure an abortion if she wished. Involvement in abortion would no longer involve *a physician's personal ethics* – these *would*, in fact, *cease*. Physicians should no longer have personal ethics. Ethics would be dictated (oh wait, I'm sure I mean to write, "be guided") by the college.

A registrar may get the message out to the readership of the monthly newsletter that if the college makes a statement, and then a physician expresses dissent to the press, he/she can be considered having committed "conduct unbecoming" a physician by having "damaged the integrity (unity) of the profession." Wow! A physician had better not express dissent, huh? Freedom of expression seems to stop at the door of the college, in the hands of certain leaders. They purvey the message: embrace company policy, or else! Such leaders have totally lost sight of how medicine has *evolved by disagreement* with one approach or opinion. It really is very healthy to be able to disagree. HSBC Bank has a current PR campaign to celebrate different points of view. Public disagreement is very Canadian!

As a part of its legislative function, a college may enact legislation just a bit too soon, without having thought through the implications of a dumb new bylaw. This is an example of the "ugly baby" syndrome. Politicians do it all the time. The new law is their "baby," and they just can't stand to have anyone acknowledge that it really is ugly. No mother wants her baby recognized as ugly – because it is a part of her. Bad legislation is like an "ugly baby" because it is a part of the proposer. But so obviously ugly that . . . everyone knows! Just like the *Emperor's New Clothes*! Transparently wrong. Yet PRIDE is involved and the *NEED to be RIGHT*! The bylaw may say that such things as cryotherapy to a wart with liquid nitrogen must be performed in an "accredited nonhospital surgical facility." Accreditation would be a process undertaken by application to the college; there would be a fee. Really, every single procedure done would require this same process. Would this be a "make-work" project? It would allow that college to employ more people, create a larger governing body? Expand its government – become a megacorporation!

Under this amazing bylaw, procedures like wart treatment and abdominal paniculectomy (tummy tuck) might be *on the same list* together – equally outlawed! It was a dumb bylaw. Eventually the college did make it more reasonable. But while it stood, at least half the family physicians in the province breached the dumb thing. With it the college could pretty easily take a bite out of anyone it disliked. It was a *BYLAW*, after all! Weird, eh? Sorry about that "eh" thing; remember, I am Canadian!

Colleges like to be self-regulating. That means that they can govern their own profession. Governance is not trivial. It is powerful. Small wonder that colleges want to continue to be "self-regulating" because that keeps the power – direct, or by influence, with them – the registrar and his *carefully selected permanent, entourage*: the buck stops there! So does the power! Some registrars might forget that they were appointed and begin to believe that they were *Anointed*! This poorly founded dogma would be called the divine right of registrars!

Within the Medical Professions Acts, under provincial, state, and federal legislation, colleges can establish bylaws. This means (as we have just discussed) that they have *legislative power*. The registrar, of course, has *executive power*. If the registrar believes that a given physician is a clear *threat to the public*, he can suspend that physician from practice. (Surprisingly, I never was. What is, logically, the reason for that – that he never did consider me a threat to the public, right?) Hearing committees, to some degree, but then the Council of the College, to its fullest, has *judicial power*. Three great powers! The French political philosopher Baron de Montesquieu described and idealized the tripartite system in which there needed to be a SEPARATION of these three powers. The independence of the power of the judiciary was to be REAL and not simply "apparent." In this instance, that means that the registrar should not control the hearings. This is to prevent *one person from wielding all three powers at once*, a potential despot – or in modern terms, a dictator or bully.

You may wonder why I use the word *bully*. Well, going through the college disciplinary system tends to catch you alone: isolate you – separate you from others, who might be colleagues or friends, but are not going through this process. Right then, it's just you going through it. You're on your own: cornered. Neighborhood bullies single their victims out too – of all of the kids at school suddenly the bully isolates one. When I was about seven years old, I was in an accelerating elementary grade situation, doing the first three grades in two years. It made me younger than my contemporaries. I also had excelled at piano, so my mom started me on the violin. Now visualize this: I was walking the three miles home from my violin lesson (so for me, music was quite aerobic). In an alleyway, the elementary school bully, whom we called Jinx, trapped me and would not let me pass. He had been held back in grade six while I was being pushed ahead. He was *much* bigger than me. He ordered me to open my violin case. I was mortified. I feared that he would break the precious violin that my parents had provided for me out of a tight budget. He plucked it out of the case, checked it out, and then . . . handed it back to me, allowing me to put it away. I was becoming hopeful, but he said, "I'm going to punch you real hard. Do you want it in the face in or the gut?" I have understood since that this was a *terrorist ploy* doubling the effect of the physical injury by preinforming me of my injury, and then requiring my choice to guide his assault. It emphasized that I had *no power whatsoever* in the situation. I had glasses, small stature, and limited family resources to replace the glasses or my violin. I chose, "The gut." Of course, he punched with all his strength. I am sure he was gratified by my crying as I walked away from him. Bullies do that! Nothing was ever done to him for the incident. However, he later did some acts of arson and, subsequently, disappeared from the school "play" ground. College proceedings, too, *give an accused no power whatsoever* in the end. I definitely felt bullied. The process of college discipline certainly does single out one from the general throng of physicians. If this is considered necessary, it behoves those "in power" to proceed very, very ethically, even gently.

Traditionally, complaints to a college would come through a patient who was dissatisfied or upset. The very purpose of the complaints department was to "give voice" to the dissatisfied or harmed patient. That was actually in the college brochure sent to doctors about whom a complaint had been made. The patient's complaint letter was copied to the physician, with that brochure, and the physician was asked to explain his or her behavior in that circumstance. An assigned member of the permanent staff of the college (assistant registrar) and an investigator would gather information, and an attempt at reconciliation would be made. That is the tradition. What I learned is that the College of Some Physicians and Surgeons can actually go out and talk to the nurses and others who may not like a physician and solicit complaints from anyone about the physician. When the college is asking about the shortcomings of a given physician, might not that actually *create* some complaints?

Also, the patient involved may actually disagree with/disapprove of the complaint. The college did this twice to me during their process of investigation. In the years of the Inquisition, this would have been called a witch hunt. Of course, the Inquisitors were just "providing ethical guidance" to the world, right – drowning or cleansing with fire by burning at the stake?

We have just been considering *overinvestigation* ("investigating" for some dirt on a physician – not "case-focused"). But does *underinvestigation* ever occur? I think so! Meaning that the specifics of the complaint might never be known until the midst of a formal disciplinary hearing, three years later [so that the information need not be DISCLOSED to the defense] – leaving the physician and his counsel no time to prepare. In my case, a very lengthy first complaint letter had been crafted by one woman, who included in the complaint letter so much incredulous and self-contradictory content, that it did not seem very difficult to defend against. This was very early in 2002. Then, another complaint was received shortly thereafter, following my having been placed on a fourteen-day suspension of privileges at their local rural hospital where I did part-time emergency work while the first complaint was being investigated for resolution. This second complaint was brief (only fourteen lines), *vague*, and seemed fairly innocuous. It was laid by the wife of the pastor to the first lady, so I certainly wanted to know more. However, *the second complainant was APPARENTLY never interviewed* by the college investigator to clarify her vague complaint. At the time of the disciplinary hearing in 2005 (THREE YEARS LATER), I *heard for the first time from her, no longer a vague complaint, but a clear description of CRIMINAL BEHAVIOR* (if physically imaginable) on my part. Was this because she simply embellished the story a bit with each fresh retelling of it over the three years, kind of like my tale of catching that really big fish? Or, had she heard from Counsel for the College that the witness/chaperone who had been with us for the exam had not been "found," so it would be *her word against mine* (so she could make her evidence as outlandish as she wished and possibly be believed)? Can you think of other explanations?

It is true that there is a legal requirement that the college supply full disclosure of any witness statements, which they have in their possession, so we must conclude as follows:

1. The college investigator just "couldn't get around to" interviewing this second lady to clarify the details of her

encounter in the ensuing three years (her week was *just too hectic* . . . for three years!).

2. The college investigator was completely and *thoroughly incompetent.*
3. A completely and thoroughly competent college investigator was *told not to interview.*
4. The college investigator *did interview*, and the results were not legally disclosed.

Those are the only reasons I could come up with. Can you think of any other possibilities? The investigator certainly *had time enough* to interview sufficient staff members from that rural hospital to find someone who could provide grounds for the college laying some other charge, unrelated to their case under investigation. The college had previously been very emphatic about my use of a chaperone. They had insisted that I use one. Doesn't it seem likely that such a chaperone would be very looked for by them, to find out what she had seen? But the investigator apparently never had the time to find the nurse/chaperone who had attended with me the second (or "me-too") complainant. Nor had she the time to interview the second complainant to clarify her exact complaint. Investigators do that, right? (From *The Long Kiss Goodnight*: "Chefs do that!") That's believable, isn't it? Oh, and the *unable-to-be-found nurse/chaperone?* Well, she was actually easily found. Imagine that? We easily identified her signature on the chart, and surprise, surprise . . . she was still working every day at that same hospital. Perhaps, in fairness, the college investigator was *no longer able to find that hospital.* The nurse in question says that *the administration DID talk with her* about that patient encounter around the time of the investigation. So maybe it was *the administrator* of the hospital who could no longer be found? Or, well . . . maybe . . . the college investigator *lost the whole darn town* in question! That can happen, right? Chefs do that! Are you starting to understand how – in my case – the power wielders in the college did not feel restrained by such petty issues as due process, ethical behavior, and fairness?

Yeah, but if a college or a hearing committee does make a blatant mistake, it can simply say, "Wait, we've made a blatant mistake! *Everyone will know* we've been unfair," can't it? Well, maybe. BUT *if they admit a mistake*, what will happen to their reputation, *their image* . . . and verily *the very fabric* of the whole profession? Oh dear, political doctors not appearing to be right! Ouch! What about the NEED to be right? So will they simply attempt to "save face"? Remember, they individually have been trained to need to be right. Will they be unethical in order to keep this *appearance*? You are going to learn that a judge from the Alberta Court of Queen's Bench believed that they could correct their mistakes. I, too, *believed that they could have*, and it really would not have damaged their image; in fact, admitting a mistake can only increase one's credibility. *They did not!*

WHO WANTS TO BE A PART OF THE COLLEGE?

There are really two aspirations: a *willingness to set aside* the joy of direct patient care part-time for a couple of years in order to make the system improve, OR a *desire to stop* doing any patient care to just be in charge of others doing patient care – a full-time bureaucrat! Who gets drawn in? Is there such a thing as a political doctor? One who is more interested in influence and sway than in patient care? This, too, might give the wrong person a chance to "get even" with the world.

No one in medicine has been to a staff, department, or association meeting without noticing a few physicians who repeatedly want to talk, who *always* proffer their ideas. Remember we said that the training and the career path engenders an "I am right!" philosophy. (I have it, too, in the writing of this book. So you are going to have to look for evidence: don't simply be swayed by my injuries or opinions.) Some who like to talk just want to talk. Others want to be heard, believed, *obeyed* . . . maybe even worshipped! There are those who really love medicine and all that it stands for. They are often willing to serve for a term of two years or so. They are not quitting medicine; they are simply trying to make medicine in their community a better place – and they do their work part-time while continuing to practice a bit less. They take a while to get rolling, and often the registrar or his associate "helps them out" – they learn to look to him for direction. After all, hasn't he given up all that they love in medicine to be the registrar. But some registrars are influence brokers.

We have learned through sad experience that it is the nature of most men, when they get a little authority (as they think), they begin to exercise unfair power or influence on others. Maybe they had been very verbal about how a certain physician who drew media attention was dealt with by the then college and expressed how *if they had "been in power"* that never would have happened. Of course, they have based their then opinion on what was printed or spoken in the media, whose very purpose is to fan the flames and focus hype – to sensationalize. The media is often not even close to accurate. However, once a given physician has vehemently spoken an opinion to his friends and colleagues, it is very human to have to hold tight to what he has said. To do otherwise would cause a loss of face. A completely unacceptable option to the political physician!

Preformed opinions are not easily influenced by new evidence. For the last ten years, there has been a movement in medicine to the concept of practicing evidence-based medicine. That means that we attempt to prove every new and all possible old methods. We seek evidence that this is the proven BEST way to treat. One of the great hurdles will be to keep up. What was the best way when you were in training may no longer be the best way just a few years later when you are in practice. This may actively thwart one of your goals as a physician: to BE RIGHT.

COMING WITH BIAS TO A DISCIPLINARY HEARING

To say that members of a given disciplinary hearing committee came with bias implies a conspiracy theory. I didn't know the committee before the hearing. Conspiracy theories are always virtually impossible to confirm or prove, even harder to prove than negligence by an expert witness. I guess that's why they are called theories. However, I think I can show you that the committee *became biased* (if it wasn't already) and perhaps *how* the members became biased.

In ordinary negligence or "not up to standards" cases, each side finds expert witnesses who provide testimony about acceptable practice. Usually they find peers of the accused. That shows that a similarly trained, similarly practicing physician, has this certain point of view. The prosecution finds a peer who says "not up to standards," and the defense finds a peer who says "seems okay by me." My defense lawyer had attempted to do just that, but the college wanted to compare me to specialists. Perhaps I should have been flattered. I wasn't, I was scared. I felt as I had when the school bully had singled me out. The college had two specialists: One was a fully trained and thirteen years practicing general surgeon. She was carefully chosen by the assistant registrar, soon-to-become registrar. He had helped to train her, and they had a long relationship. He knew her views, her outspokenness: he hired a "hit man"! She certainly was not a peer. She'd have been about forty-seven years old but was petite and a "handsome figure of a woman." She could hold the gaze of the two older male panelists pretty easily. And what of the third panelist: the nonphysician, social worker? Well, the registrar secretly knew that she venerated women of power – like a female surgeon competing with the best of the male surgeons (in a totally male-dominated field). Dr. DDDD spoke forcefully, passionately, convincingly. If I had not myself been the accused, I'd have stood up and applauded after her soliloquies, *as I would after any other actress.* I think I saw the social worker (clearly the woman's fan) genuflecting a few times. We were enthralled. We were entranced. We were . . . *played!* And the then assistant registrar sat there and did his half-smile of triumph. He did not rein in his protégée – did not demand of her the balance, fairness, and impartiality required of an expert witness. As producer and director of this little production, he had won. He knew it! *Wow, was he special!* With regard to breast exam, my lawyer got a fellow family physician and *real peer* to speak as an expert in my behalf. He was able to confirm what was accepted in the community, but he was certainly less glitzy than the female surgeon, who specialized in breast surgery. It certainly appeared that we were outgunned!

There were two things wrong with the assistant registrar's approach though:

1. He had compared my practice methods to those of an accomplished surgeon. "Ah, but wait," chimed in his legal watchdog. "My view [and therefore the paramount legal view here – remember he believes he is the prosecutor, the legal advisor to the college, *and the judge!*] is that because Dr. DDDD occasionally lectures to medical students and residents, even groups of family doctors, her practice must be the standard against which Litchfield should be measured!"

2. AND *his prize pupil,* the standard against whom all physicians everywhere should be compared, and now his mouthpiece who had spoken so eloquently against me, *was wrong* . . . in several instances!

Are you becoming a bit more curious? How could a "less right" (family) physician say that about a "more right *special* (-ist) *physician*"?

The second witness for the college was a trained doctor of osteopathy. He was the first DO registered by the College of Physicians and Surgeons of Alberta although they have been around for years in the States. He was an Alberta "pilot project" if you will. He was under careful scrutiny by the college because some of what he did looked an awful lot like chiropractic stuff. I got the sense from him that he was desperately trying to be truthful. I did not feel under attack by him. That was because he actually did understand and stick to his actual role in the judicial system as an expert witness. Counsel for the College certainly did try to "sic" him on me, but I did not feel venom from his mouth. I was to be compared against him with regard to manual therapy. And I certainly did feel that he was the better trained of the two of us in that regard. He is more qualified and better trained than I. He is not a peer either. Again, counsel focused on his qualifications to speak about manual therapy because he was licensed as a family doctor and was a preceptor to some family medicine residents. He was a part of the Department of Family Practice at the University of Calgary, my former alma mater. He was up and coming. I was to be compared to him. I have to admit that I envy him his training.

We are both members of the Canadian Association of Orthopaedic Medicine (CAOM). I see him at conferences. I know he has learned well. Anticipating the involvement of the osteopath, my lawyer secured the services of my teacher and mentor Dr. Donald Fraser of St. Catherines, Ontario, who also practices in Lewiston, New York, and had been chairman of orthopedic medicine in Rochester, New York. He had been doing manual medicine for many years – from before the osteopath had been born. This time, the Counsel for the College attempted to discredit him by saying that he hadn't been doing family medicine for many years, so of what worth would his opinion on manual therapy technique be? To dismiss the opinion of the older, more experienced physician seems trivial to you, counsel. *Have you never learned respect* for those who have amassed so much knowledge? Do you do that within the legal profession as well?

Now you may need to stop reading here and think about this incongruity. My mentor, a very experienced practitioner of manual medicine, has an opinion that should be given less weight in my hearing because he *no longer* actively practices full family medicine. But the college's breast surgical expert has an opinion that should be given greater weight in my hearing in spite of her having *never* practiced family medicine. At the very least, this thinking is inconsistent. More likely, it's unfair. Well, or helping to define "ethical guidance" to the profession.

WHO WANTS TO BE AN EXPERT WITNESS?

We began with the premise that physicians like to think they are right! So there are some naturally alluring aspects to being a medical expert witness. Just having the medical community recognize your rightness is pretty heady stuff. Dropping the comment at a social gathering that you have to be an expert witness in a hearing or court case next week can certainly earn some brownie points. It feels good. Maybe we should ask the question, *Who doesn't want to be an expert medical witness?* Here, the doctors and their main reasons are more obvious. Those that don't want to be called as expert witnesses tend to be those that aren't sure if they are right and don't want to shed light on their shortcomings. There may be some other reasons, but not many. However, a very good one would be to decline this positive recognition – if the apparent duties compromised a physician's personal principles. College expert witnesses certainly get paid very well for their time. They become part of the college's inner circle [if you don't know what this means, talk to someone who has practiced for more than ten years].

How does the college choose its experts? They make a list of physicians of good reputation and good language skills, but is good repute enough? No, they send a file and ask for the potential inner circle candidate's opinion. *This is important!* If you review the file and provide an opinion that does not match their expectation, they may send you back the file and ask for another review; OR, *they may never send you another file!* That means you're not going to be one of the insiders. If you're new in the province, state, territory, or jurisdiction [or if you are the first, say, registered osteopath in the province], then you are going to feel all the more pressure to provide the "sought" opinion. Also true if you've ever had trouble with the college before, and they have a noose on you. And if you feel some pride in your accomplishments and think you've not been adequately recognized for all your knowledge, you might just bend a bit. You can justify biased testimony by saying that you are just providing a clear opinion on one side of the issue. After all, they have their defense lawyers, don't they? Those lawyers ought to enable the provision of the other side of the issue, right? So it's *OK to not quite provide the whole truth* under oath. Thinking that will probably salve your conscience somewhat, at least.

However, there are actual published standards. The American College of Surgeons has provided recommended guidelines for behavior of the physician acting as an expert witness. Here are three of seven:

1. Physicians have an obligation to testify in court as expert witnesses when appropriate. Physician expert witnesses are expected to be *impartial and should not adopt a position as an advocate or partisan in the legal proceedings.*

2. The physician expert witness should review all the relevant medical information in the case and testify to its content *fairly, honestly, and in a balanced manner.* In addition, the physician expert witness may be called upon to draw an inference or an opinion based on the facts of the case. In doing so, the physician expert witness should apply the *same standards of fairness and honesty.*

3. (There are actually a 3, 4, 5, and 6, but I'm skipping right to number 7 so I don't bore you.) The physician expert witness is *ethically and legally obligated to tell the truth.* TRANSCRIPTS of depositions and courtroom testimony are public records and subject to independent peer reviews. Moreover, the physician expert witness should willingly provide transcripts and other documents pertaining to the expert testimony to independent peer review if requested by his or her professional organization. The physician expert witness should be aware that *failure to provide truthful* testimony exposes the physician expert witness to *criminal prosecution* for perjury, civil suits for negligence, and revocation or suspension of his or her professional license.

AN EXPERT WITNESS IN CANADA

Of course, I live in Canada. What is expected of an expert witness in Canada? From *Canada Gazette* Vol. 143, No. 42 – October 17, 2009, we read as follows:

"A number of jurisdictions, including the Federal Court, have identified potential concerns with respect to the current approach to expert testimony before the Courts, in particular with respect to the independence of Experts. The misapprehension of the role of expert witnesses in the trial process can result in *experts advocating on behalf of a party.*" [No, no! Say it ain't so. Could that actually happen, here?] "*Such an approach diminishes the reliability and usefulness of the expert's evidence* to the Court." Therefore, the "Rules Committee has developed a number of amendments to give Judges the tools they require to ensure that expert evidence is adduced in the most efficient, least costly and <u>fairest</u> manner." [Actually, I added the underlining on the word *fairest*, just so you know.]

This document goes on to explain how <u>Proposed new rule 52.2</u> "requires counsel to provide an expert witness with a copy of the Code of Conduct and to file a certificate signed by the expert acknowledging that the expert agrees to be bound by the Code of Conduct."

Now, my lawyer did provide a real peer physician to me. This was Dr. David Brown, a family physician. He maintained the exact balance of fairness and lack of bias required of an expert witness and, when asked for an opinion, provided it. But he wasn't necessarily exciting because he didn't enter into the fray. And he wasn't as glitzy as the college's nonpeer surgical specialist. He confirmed my practices of technique in breast exam and abdominal exam from a family physician's standard. Yet he didn't take sides – he just gave his views. So what do you think, M. le Registrar? Do you think an impartial *real judge* would figure that your expert and protégé might possibly have "advocated on behalf of a party," you? And what might Mr. or Mdm. Justice think about her also *being less than truthful under oath and suppressing evidence from the very article from which she quoted*? Impartial, balanced, and fair? Those seem the goals for expert witnesses. Their absence caused me great personal sadness and pain. There seemed to be no avenue of recourse for the unfairness – do I appeal to the very panel of judges that is bending the rules?

ARE EXPERT WITNESSES EXPERTS IN EVERYTHING?

Years ago, television ad testimonials were done by celebrities. That person didn't have to be an expert in soap, soup, cars, or breakfast cereal. He or she did the ad because they were paid. They were popular figures, but not experts. So what about medical "expert witnesses"? Are they experts in everything, or should they stick to exactly what their expertise is in?

Should an expert witness adopt a position of advocacy? Should *they* try to be lawyers (in French: *avocats*)? Should they actually argue the case? Should they anticipate the arguments of the actual lawyers and attempt to outlawyer them? No, that would show bias! *BUT* one expert in "all diseases of the breast" did. An example of her legal argument would be on page 335, lines 9 and on: "If you're making the argument . . ." And page 336, lines 2-5, in answering the question "the fact that a woman is able to breast feed does not by itself rule out a problem with one of those ducts, right?" To which she takes over the questioning by asking, "What kind of problems would you be envisioning?" Page 360, lines 12 and 13, she questions the lawyer further and defiantly with, "What would he possibly find on the pelvic examination on the second day that he didn't find the first day?" So what do you think, l'Expert? Do you think that these readers will pretty well know that you came with a bias – a position of advocacy?

Counsel for the College did get a very repetitive commitment to her position on this attempting to express secretions from the nipple in the course of a routine physical exam of the breast:

1. He: "And I think you were very clear [re: nipple expression] that there was no purpose." (p. 372)

2. He: "Do you know of any school of thought that would recommend it?"
   L'Expert: "It is only spontaneous, unilateral, bloody discharge that you would worry about." (also p. 269)

3. He: "I think you've already said that compression between finger and thumb is not a part of a regular breast exam." (p. 273)

4. He: "Is there any information from your <u>literature review</u> . . . that lends support to that method of examination [expression] being a current method or, at least in 2001, a current method of examination?"
   L'Expert: "Not at all!" (p. 368)

This sets out her evidence pretty clearly: she has not simply relied on her own knowledge but claims to have done a 'search of the literature; and, finds no source would agree with my practice approach. Are you with me?

EXPERT WITNESS TAKES SIDES IS UNTRUTHFUL

Then both lawyers question her about the textbook that I had used to demonstrate to the patient involved that nipple expression WAS a part of a routine examination. Page 328, lines 9-15:

L'Expert: "It [the Novey text] gives the detailed examination of the breast."

My lawyer: And it doesn't say anywhere in there that you should only do this if you have elicited a history of discharge. Correct?

L'Expert: (*In not answering the question*) "And what I'm saying is I suspect if you look at any part of this book, *it doesn't tell you the circumstances under which you do each part* of a physical examination, but ..."

My lawyer: (Trying to focus her attention on a contradiction in the very thing that she has just said that, *in fact, it does tell you the circumstances under which you do this further part* of a physical examination) "Well, if we look, in fact, at the next point, it talks about additional things you should do if discharge is seen or suspected, *which suggests that you attempt routinely to express discharge ...*"

Now the "expert" feigns obtuseness here, so my lawyer gives the question to her in a different package (p. 329): "So point one gives an unqualified recommendation as to what you should do in an exam. Point two sets out additional things you should do if discharge is seen or suspected from history. That's correct?" And again, L'Expert demonstrates she is not here to be honest, fair, unbiased, or balanced in her evidence – by [again] not answering the question, this time by attempting to *redirect* the focus of questioning [Mme L'Expert, have you ever had any children? Teenagers? This redirection is what they always do when they are losing an argument with a parent]. She does this by stating, "It would be very . . . um . . . *I would be interested in the publication date* that would say that."

Oops, Expert 1! That's unfortunate. What did you just say? *Why would the publication date be important,* Mme L'Expert? When you were questioned about an apparent difference between your prehearing statements about older techniques and your evidence under oath, you said [*under oath*] that you had just been generously giving me "the benefit of the doubt." Then you've stated that, in fact, *no source [not even an outdated source] recommended the checking of the nipple for expressible secretions* in the course of a routine breast exam. No source! So *why ask your question about the date,* Mme L'Expert? Did you know that some authorities of older date did, in fact, recommend this? Readers might think that you were lying under oath here. Oops! Why would you do that to me? Did the registrar know? Or *did you do it all by yourself?* Were you told that Dr. Litchfield would be financially destroyed and would never have the time or means to reassess your statements? He'd be too busy as an old man just trying to get a job or jobs to earn a living for his family after he was bankrupted by the college and his license to practice [livelihood] had been taken away, right? Or he'd certainly have to leave the country to practice in a third world country. No one would ever be around to tell the world that *you had not only lied, but been caught in a lie,* right? Had you been provided reassurances? Or, did you act all on your own? If so, why?

Further excerpts from the official transcript of my disciplinary hearing and the findings of the hearing committee are here provided to terrify and enlighten you: this is a very serious business. And the PEER Physician did get it right!

BREAST EXAM AND FINDINGS: Their expert says she possesses *knowledge of all diseases of the breast:* Page 260: "I lecture to the medical students and to residents of many of the specialties. I have lectured to family physicians as well regarding BOTH benign and malignant (breast) disease." This is to emphasize how knowledgeable she is.

Then, to show how little knowledge I have in comparison, she states, "I think if you ask 100 physicians, and you are the

Only one doing it that way – then it is inappropriate" (p. 316). She acknowledges that she has not, in fact, asked one hundred physicians. So why the phrase? Well, it is again to make seem more correct one's opinion. It adds no new evidence but is used by a witness who is showing that her evidence is better than someone else's [Remember the issue of competition and neutrality of an expert witness?].

Is her statement intrinsically true? If you ask one hundred physicians and you are the only one doing it that way, then is it inappropriate? Could it not also be that you know something that even a majority doesn't? While attending the American Academy of Family Physicians national scientific assembly, I attended a workshop with Jeff Unger, director of the Chino California Headache Center. He asked the more than fifty of the assembled physicians how many of the attendees knew how to assess the occipital nerves as a cause of headaches. Guess how many hands went up? Only mine! So *is that inappropriate?* Guess again, Ms. Expert.

WAYS OF TRAINING A DOCTOR

I understand the college expert attended medical school at the University of Alberta. She certainly developed some allegiance to a surgeon who later became registrar during her residency program in surgery in Edmonton. However, I think it is very important to just focus on the accusations against me and how they were handled by the registrar and those whom he recruited. The facts are that she did medical school in Edmonton and then did a brief internship in Calgary. She then returned to Edmonton to do her surgical residency then a one-year ICU residency in Edmonton. So she really doesn't have any training outside Alberta. The fact that she did surgical residency in Edmonton, in part, under the "ethical guidance" of the "registrar before he was" and was now his prize witness, I will just have to live with. However, these things we know. She went to medical school in Edmonton, a traditional medical school. And she says that *she continues to do her breast and abdominal exams just the same way that she had learned in medical school.*

After my master's degree in experimental surgery in Edmonton, I also went to medical school in Alberta – in Calgary, a nontraditional medical school. In the first few weeks of medical school, it is easy to feel overwhelmed by the volume of material for which you are about to become responsible. And – now this is important – in Calgary we were taught – you students are *responsible for acquiring* all that it is to be a competent physician. You can go to classes or not. But you need to learn all there is to becoming competent doctors. We (the faculty) will *help* you achieve your goal! But it is you students who must do it! *Always acquire more than one approach or opinion.* The first one may be incorrect. Build your knowledge of medicine by having many sources – many teachers, many books, and many preceptors – so that you can glean the truth (or your best approximation to it).

I was married already and had two wonderful children – the older, a two-year-old. As I studied at a desk at home, I often held one on each knee while my wife curled up into a little ball near my feet and slept. The rule was that if the children talked much, they couldn't stay on my lap. That was the harsh reality: I needed lots of time and an environment that allowed me to concentrate. I had to make every moment count. For the formal study time at a desk or a table early in my training in physical exam, I often used a recommended textbook by Barbara Bates; it was large and required a desktop surface to lay it out. But I also learned (second source) that there were precious minutes in the day that I would be waiting for a preceptor (teaching doctor) waiting for a class to start, waiting for some costudents to arrive for a study/review group, or during lunches. And in these minutes I poured over a brown softcover (and small enough to fit in my medical student jacket pocket) also recommended textbook called *Bedside Diagnostic Examination* by DeGowin and DeGowin, third edition and published in 1976 (and I was using it from the year I started in 1979). Dr. Janet Wright, who is now a permanent part of the college in my province and former classmate, could confirm this. When I saw my psychiatrist on Monday, March 8, 2010, he told me he, too, had used this as his learning text and had it sitting right on his shelf! His brown softcover copy felt so comfortable in my hand. This textbook gave a more practical application, it seemed, than the Bates text. For example, in the section on the female breast, on page 249, I found "Examination of the Nipples. No special posture of the patient is required. Inspect the skin of the anterior trunk for supernumerary [extra] nipples. Look for retraction of the nipple; ascertain whether the deformity is recent or old; recent ones suggest acquired disease. Look for fissures in the nipples. *Search for discharge from the nipples by gently compressing the nipple and areola between the thumb and forefinger*, note the color of the discharge." [My note: There were no caveats such as, "Only do this if there has been a complaint of spontaneous discharge." It was just describing part of a complete breast exam!] "Look for dry scaling and red excoriation of the nipple. Palpate the periphery of the areola for tender nodules." The book next explored the medical considerations of any of the findings on nipple examination, such as the bilateral discharge of galactorrhea, the unilateral discharge of possible duct pathology, and the diseases with which an eczematous nipple can be associated. It was so logically written and enlightening. I was thrilled with it as a sound reference, and I was very committed to following its direction exactly. And I have done so. *Doesn't this sound like what L'Expert 1 says is NOT a part of the breast exam?*

FOREGONE CONCLUSIONS

L'Expert says that *after her extensive literature search* (page 265, line 26 and on) *in NONE of the literature* "do they state that you should express the nipple, especially in the absence of a nipple complaint" (page 266 lines 3–8). This committee, of course, allowed that *she must be expert also in "all of the literature"* – like the tennis champion talking about the best possible soap! What a horrid mistake! She only used one source in learning physical exam, and it is (unfortunately) still the main recommended source book for physical exam at her school, the University of Alberta. The attendant at the health sciences area of the UofA Bookstore says that for some reason, the Bates book is the virtually exclusive recommendation, and all the little students buy just what they are told. It's tradition. And yet there may be more than four hundred alternatives (on AllBookstores.com). You will want to read my chapter on printed methods of physical examination (in chapter 9) very carefully. I promise it will be enlightening.

Having the expert's bias allows her to superimpose her prejudgement on a text (like the one by Don Novey in 1990) with which she is unfamiliar and say, "HE MEANS *you would only express if there was a specific complaint of spontaneous discharge*, and here's how you would do it." Woe, now! The actual CONSIDERATION of the importance of spontaneous nipple discharge (SND) only came into the medical literature *five to eight years AFTER he wrote his book*. So I guess . . . maybe he was *clairvoyant* too, huh? Obviously, the history of medicine is not within your expert knowledge. You really should have met Dr. Peter Cruise, a surgeon from Calgary. He was fascinating in his description and awareness of the history of medicine: how did we get to where we are now? His knowledge certainly did command my respect. But wait, he was older then, so maybe his opinion would be given less weight by the committee, right?

In fairness to this frightfully naïve expert, her training ended and her practice began in 1992. Year 1995 was about when an interest in spontaneous nipple discharge (SND) began to be present in the literature: Dunn et al. says in the *British Journal of Surgery* (Remember, the *expert is a surgeon*. Have you heard of this journal, Mme L'Expert?), 1995 Jun; 82(6):789–91: "All patients with expressible or spontaneous nipple discharges and those with skin changes at the nipple should undergo examination of cytological smears." Of course, this examination of cytological smears is the very thing that I had been doing with such specimens. The noble disciplinary hearing committee *criticized and ridiculed me* about it. Their expert's view is that only *spontaneous AND unilateral* discharge (plus or minus, bloody) can be viewed to be pathological. She is emphatic about that. Well . . . she is emphatic about everything.

The idea of SND versus expressible or evoked nipple discharge (END) was actually argued back and forth in the literature for years. Somewhat more recently, Vargas HI et al. in the article "Outcomes of Clinical and Surgical Assessment of Women with Pathological Nipple Discharge," Am Surg (Oh, and *this too would be the surgical, not family practice, literature*) 2006 February 72(2):124–8, describes pathological nipple discharge (no longer END or SND but PND) as *unilateral in 96 percent, bloody* in 79 percent, and *spontaneous in 62 percent.* Spontaneous in 62 percent! That means 38 percent of pathologic nipple discharges are not spontaneous. Expert for the college, are you satisfied with *missing 38 percent of pathological nipple discharge* by your bias that if the patient doesn't complain of it (spontaneous), then it can't be pathological? Do your patients know that you are missing about four out of ten of them? Do you think they would like to be informed? Oh, by the way, the Vargas Group is at the Harbor-UCLA Medical Center in Torrance, California. I think they might practice kinda good medicine there. You might want to not just stay in Alberta but get out and do some CME there and elsewhere.

CASTING ASPERSIONS

For some reason the expert looked up and decided to borrow evidence from an article by Monica Morrow from the *Journal of the American Academy of Family Physicians.* This is her second unethical action against me. I suspect that she wanted to insult me with literature from my own discipline (family practice). She *quoted from it extensively, but she also failed to quote important aspects of the very article* to the panel/committee. *By doing so, she misled the committee* by her spin on the quotes. Page 269 of the transcripts, line 18 gives her view: "Nipple discharge is frequently yellow or green, dark [as opposed to bloody]. That is normal physiologic discharge." But Dr Monica Morrow says that three factors other than an obvious bloody look, would make the discharge possibly pathologic: they being – 1. found only on one side [one-sidedness]; 2. associated with a mass; OR, 3. associated with microscopic blood."

Another example of her carrying her bias to this situation is from this same article: "Because stimulation of the nipple (i.e., squeezing to check for discharge) actually promotes discharge, patients with a *physiologic* discharge should be advised to avoid checking for discharge." May I add that I totally agree with this counsel if given to an *overly zealous patient with a physiologic discharge.*

However, the key for the physician is to determine not just *whether the discharge is present, but whether it is physiologic*! But the expert says, "Well, if patients shouldn't check, then physicians shouldn't either!" Did she really say that? Oh my! That kind of puts you out on a limb, Ms. Expert! Now is that the same as claiming, "Well, if patients shouldn't check five times a day for the *presence* of discharge, then physicians shouldn't determine once a year [at the annual medical] the *nature* of whatever discharge is present"? Is there some "only known to her" logic here (transcripts on page 332)? More importantly, she *failed to disclose* that in the Monica Morrow article in American Family Physician that the lawyer for the college introduced "in its entirety" as exhibit no. 4, page 2,373, there is other important guidance:

> "The first step in the evaluation of a nipple discharge is to *determine whether the discharge is pathologic or physiologic.* Nipple discharges are classified as pathologic if they are 1. spontaneous, 2. bloody, or 3. associated with a mass. Pathologic discharges are usually, 4. *unilateral* and, 5. *confined to one duct.* Physiologic discharges are characterized by 1. discharge only with compression and by 2. multiple duct involvement . . . , frequently 3. *bilateral.*" So there are these five characteristics that describe pathologic discharges [I added the numbers] and three that describe physiologic [no real medical problem] discharges. The presence of a pathologic discharge does NOT mean that there is cancer, of course, just some kind of pathologic process. But why did the expert raise some parts of this article and fail to raise these others? From whom is she withholding information? Her evidence certainly harmed me. And it was jaded.

Can you see how Dr. Morrow did not pursue the college expert's overarching simplification: "*Nipple discharges are classified as pathologic, only if they are spontaneous. Physiologic discharges are characterized by discharge only with compression.*" Such a view would have certainly been easier, but it would not be accurate, and Dr. Morrow wanted to be ACCURATE. She's a surgeon, Mme L'Expert, but *she's not like you*, is she?

Then on page 2,374 of her journal article, Dr. Morrow states, "The workup of a pathologic discharge should include localization of the affected duct and examination of the discharge for occult blood. Cytology generally is not useful [so here, in her 2000 article, Monica disagrees with the Dunn method recommended in 1995 in the *British Journal of Surgery*, and which I was still using] because *the absence of malignant cells does not exclude cancer, and a positive result cannot distinguish intraductal cancer from invasive cancer*." Now, in fairness, I had been doing cytology with the hope that the lab would *also* report blood cells. But then I phoned Monica Morrow, the author of this article, and asked her *how she tested* for occult blood. She told me that she uses a Hemoccult kit like what we use for screening the stool of patients with a possibility of colon cancer.

Recognizing me as a family physician, she also emphasized the next paragraph in her April 2000 article: "*All patients with 1. spontaneous, OR 2. unilateral nipple discharge, should be referred for surgical evaluation.* [Now, dear reader, you can easily count the number of criteria she is listing here, right? There are <u>two</u> criteria emphasized for referral!] This is true for patients with bloody discharges and for those with clear or serous discharges [both possibly pathological]. A terminal duct excision is both diagnostic and, for discharges that turn out to have a benign cause, therapeutic."

So why did the expert fail to disclose Dr. Morrow's full evidence? True, the spontaneous discharge idea *could be* communicated in answer to historic questioning, and this is probably the reason for her criticism of me – that I was looking for discharge but not asking about it. BUT the *unilateral discharge could only be found by checking each breast for discharge on physical exam*, and finding it on one side but not the other! In my exams, I did not ask about the presence of spontaneous nipple discharge because I knew that I always checked each breast for it. Please note that Dr. Monica Morrow refers to terminal duct excision as being therapeutic for the benign causes, and by implication . . . *there can be nonbenign causes – cancer*! And nipple expression that might help find that cancer is something the college expert says is *more than just unnecessary*: "It is inappropriate!" repeatedly, and "so now why are you doing it?" (page 335). She even goes on to say that "if I were doing breast compression and saw a [unilateral] discharge that she [the patient] hadn't noticed, I wouldn't do anything more. It's physiologic" (page 322).

That's certainly not what Dr. Morrow would suggest. BUT perhaps *no one would dare to say that you had acted improperly* because you are, after all, a friend to the registrar and *an "expert" . . . even if you neglect signs of cancer!*

So this left me wondering why the expert witness was so biased, knowing that her testimony would harm me. Had I done harm to her at any time? This is so painful. Why had I merited her compromising her medical ethics to cause me harm? She was a professional of consequence and simply aligned herself against me, my livelihood, and my family. Why was she passionate in her disdain for me? I knew her words condemned me but didn't *know why she was willing* to change her testimony, speak falsely against me, and withhold the part of the Monica Morrow article that de-vilified me. For several nights after her testimony, I slept poorly. I had the scriptures on my night table and Viktor Frankl's book *The Meaning of Life* and read them in the night. Jesus Christ was a wise teacher with a divine nature who willingly did not survive political persecution; Victor was a survivor of life in a Nazi concentration camp, hence, my holocaust theme. I became inwardly aware of their methods: choosing to be happy and helpful during a situation of oppression. I felt such a weight on my own heart that I needed help. My profession was less noble than I had thought. But I had given so much of myself to it. Indeed, I slept little those nights, and I began to lose my appetite.

COMMITTEE INFERS WRONGFULNESS

The disciplinary hearing committee found (based on her incorrect testimony) sinisterness and an invasion of the patient's rights to sexual privacy on my part, hence, grounds for them finding me guilty of unbecoming conduct by a physician. This seems to be what gave them their irrefutable moral certitude. But *what about the very article* introduced into evidence? Did the committee ever even read it? Or did they just take the information on the expert's say so? Had she simply convinced them and they were otherwise faultless?

Well, yes, *we know they did read it because they misquoted from it in their findings*: Findings page 10: "The article affirms that pathologic discharge is spontaneous, and anyone with that should be referred to a surgeon for evaluation." *Oops, committee, the expert did not say that* in her evidence. So that wasn't you just quoting her. The closest source for that statement came from Monica Morrow's article itself: "All patients with spontaneous or unilateral nipple discharge should be referred for surgical evaluation." So they, THE COMMITTEE, read the article and *intentionally dropped the words "or unilateral"* [one-sided]. Why is that? Did all members of the committee read the article, and did they jointly *collude to exclude that "unilateral discharge" evidence*, or was one of them assigned or volunteered to read the article and report back to the committee? Possibly just one of them was "playing" the others. So, committee, which of you subverted the evidence: the family doctor, the pediatrician, or the social worker? Or did you join hands and do it together? In the movie *Shawshank Redemption*, the character played by Tim Robbins refers to the warden as completely obtuse. Is that your defense? Do you claim complete obtuseness: *you just didn't know* what you were excluding? Or, were you just demonstrating *how to provide "ethical guidance* to the profession," the physicians of Alberta? Do you think you have fairly represented the ethics of the majority of Alberta doctors in excluding this evidence? Will they be happy to inform doctors from elsewhere of their pride in college committees? *What a tragedy, you three will forever be used as an example of unethical behavior by a college disciplinary committee!* Do you think you merit what you have gained by pleasing the registrar?

Samuel T. Coleridge wrote in 1802:

> How seldom, friend, a good great man inherits
> Honour or wealth, with all his worth and pains!
> It sounds like stories from the land of spirits

If any man obtain that which he merits,
Or any merit that which he obtains.

The panel's findings continue on page 12: "It has been established, as factual, that Dr Litchfield's pattern of practice in examining a woman's breast involves an effort to express secretions from the nipples despite no patient complaints. The Panel had *grave concerns over the motivation of this doctor* for performing this maneuver on a patient for no clinically relevant purpose [that we know of]. This patient felt violated by the doctor and complained. He has unjustifiably incorporated a clinical maneuver to camouflage a *sinister act* conducted in a professional atmosphere. We find his conduct unbecoming a physician."

Then, in reference to Don Novey's *Rapid Access Guide to Physical Exam*, which the committee referred to as "the article which was shown to the patient" as diagrammatically showing the technique of breast examination and the technique of expressing nipples for secretions. (Our expert) "interpreted the intent of the textbook was to teach technique only and made a point that there was no text to support a purpose to performing this maneuver. She suggested the only time this technique should be used would be when there was a history of spontaneous discharge and the duct in question should be located for diagnostic probing." Again, *they relied on her false information* to find me guilty. And they were fast asleep when my (then) lawyer got her to ask "I would, er, uhm . . . when was that book published?" after she had denied her assertion that the technique had once been published. And now, *YOU know more* than that fine committee did. You may, in fact, also be more ethical than they. And that is painful to me because I had chosen medicine as the best, most excellent career. I expected the best, most excellent colleagues. My peers!

BREAST-FEEDING ISSUES: With comments by the surgeon.

"The ducts must have been functioning properly if she is breast feeding successfully."

"*If you have plugging of a duct* that is of any importance, *then you develop mastitis*, WHICH IS A PAINFUL, RED BREAST" (page 336). So any stage before the painful red breast is unimportant? I did present evidence to describe how to treat plugged (epithelialized) ducts (white blebs) in lines 15–19 of page 518.

"You know, *mastitis is a red breast.* It is not subtle," says the expert (page 337). [At least she's consistent in her wrongness.] Just hold on there, lady, you're talkin' up your favorite soup and soap. *Breast-feeding is not what you're an expert in.* As a paragon of ethics, shouldn't you just say, "That is not my field"? Jan Riordan (*Breastfeeding and Human Lactation*) and Ruth Lawerence (*Breastfeeding: A Guide for the Medical Profession*), who are real experts in this area, would have to disagree with you about mastitis being a red breast. They would concur with Helene Cantlie in Canadian Family Physician [Remember the college expert's misdirection to the disciplinary hearing committee was based on something from the American Family Physician, which I have said actually did contain true information, so maybe even "experts" can learn from mere family practice journals, which *an arrogant type of surgeon* might think was beneath her or him.] Vol. 34, October 1988, "Treatment of Acute Puerperal Mastitis and Breast Abscess" says on page 2,222: "Histologically, mastitis [my insert: Helene is talking about *bacterial* mastitis] can be classified in three categories: cellulitis, adenitis, and breast abscess. Cellulitis involves the mammary connective tissue. In adenitis, the milk ducts are infected, and in breast abscess the infection has become encapsulated." Of course, <u>only the cellulitis shows the "red breast"</u> sign, Mme L'Expert. All *real experts* in this area know that in doing your routine breast exam with nipple expression on a nursing mom with *just subtle symptoms or signs,* an adenitis can be discovered by *seeing PUS coming from one of the ducts of a nonred breast.* And it requires attention *before* it becomes an abscess. Madam L'Expert, just face it; *you are NOT an expert* in this area of nonmalignant breast disease, even if the panel figured you were, as you claimed, an expert in "ALL diseases of the breast." The gaps in your knowledge may cause physical harm to patients, as it has caused professional and emotional harm to me.

She also says (page 269), "If the patient comes in specifically complaining about nipple discharge, and even with that, you would want a more detailed history before you would worry about it. If they have bilateral nipple discharge, it's normal." Come, now, this is *certainly* not true. In the nonpregnant nonnursing woman, galactorrhea (breast discharge from both breasts) may be the first signal of a prolactin-secreting tumor in the brain. Of this, the college expert is also undoubtedly aware; but she is on a mission, an assignment, and so *failed to provide the whole truth under oath.*

She comments on my notation of redness around the nipple by saying, "It sounds to me like surface erythema [redness], and he put her on a cream for it" (blissful ignorance? page 339). Is that cream, then, a "take-away-redness cream" [an industrial term] or some other type? If the "expert" had simply read the chart, she would have learned that in the absence of pus coming out of one duct or an obvious duct occlusion/epithelialization, I was treating nipple yeast infection (also called yeast mastitis) with an ANTIFUNGAL cream! Yet she has characterized herself as an expert in "ALL diseases of the breast" (page 259, line 27).

THE COMMITTEE INFERS, AGAIN

The committee, on page 13, stated with regard to this issue that I "cited that there was a peri-nipple redness that he thought significant of a yeast irritation [misquoted: what the heck is a *yeast irritation*, panelists? Are you just inventing new terms as you go along?], but did not suggest there were any signs of mastitis." *So this committee also doesn't know what "yeast mastitis" in a lactating mother is* and would not know how to treat it if they did find it. But wait, *there is a pediatrician* as one of the panelists! Surely, he would know that infant oral thrush (yeast) can be concomitant with maternal nipple yeast infection (not a bacterial but a yeast mastitis). Is it even remotely possible that he hasn't ever treated infantile "thrush" (oral yeast) in his years of pediatric practice? Or rather – in terms that *this* panel can understand – an oral yeast *IRRITATION?*

They then go on to say, (page 14 of findings), "*The Testimony and written submissions from [the College Expert whose name I am withholding) was felt to be reflective of the standard of care that would hold for all physicians in all areas of practice.*" In other words, they relied on her evidence (although it was wrong) and feel that it should be binding on all physicians everywhere! Wow! They further concluded that "given his pattern of breast exam which he admits involve nipple stimulation routinely, no proof of any clinical relevance, a *sinister pattern of behaviour* has been established to the panel. There is a *sexual boundary crossing* in his actions and the panel finds his conduct unbecoming a physician."

So things that enable diagnoses that you panelists are unable to make or to comprehend must be sexual boundary crossings? Either you (1) don't know much medicine, or you have (2) just been totally hoodwinked by the expert and the assistant registrar, OR you (3) knowingly proceeded unethically. Which was it, team?

ABDOMINAL EXAM AND IMPORTANCE OF OVARIES: Also with comments from the (expert) surgeon!

"I'm not actually sure I know what he thought [Does she *usually* know what others are thinking?] was happening . . ." (page 290).

"I have absolutely no idea of why WE did a pelvic examination at all!" (page 293). This medical "we" is the center of some very good medical humor. The nurse says to the patient, "Good morning, how did we sleep last night? Do we have any pain? Have we eaten all of our breakfast? Did we have our shower this morning? It is time for your enema!" Well, medical humor, you know.

The college expert continues, "I don't know what causes of right lower quadrant pain he was looking for, especially since all of his conclusions are that this is a GI complaint" (page 301).

"When it [the expert's source book] talks about the right lower quadrant pain, it has five different diagnoses that sort of come before anything [page 301 continued] gynaecologic, and the gynaecologic ones they talk of are"

1. pelvic inflammatory disease,
2. ectopic pregnancy, and
3. ovarian cyst rupture.

"You would require a gynaecologic history if you were going to do a gynaecological [exam]" (page 345–346). [The expert's assumption here is that no gynecologic history was available for review from the page in my chart just before the current one, from when she had her most recent complete medical. This is certainly one of the difficulties using a surgical specialist to criticize a family doctor – they just don't know what we do in providing care. Looking at the previous page on the chart that contains a *full* record of the patient's most recent complete medical is something no surgical specialist would ever think of accessing because they don't ever do complete medicals on patients to create a database. And she goes on to describe its very usefulness:] "I don't know if most people would remember . . . what had happened a month before," she says (page 348). I happen to agree with her on this point. *I would not remember such things, but I took great notes right at the time* [not later with a bottle of wine], and this patient's summary of the last complete medical was on the page just previous. I always made those last complete medical summary pages face forward in the chart so that I could easily refer to them. I could easily say, "Well, we did a complete medical on you just one month ago [and while referring to the summary] has anything in your [gynaecologic] history changed?" And list specific things.

The expert says, "What would he possibly find . . ." – (page 360) – "if you're looking for a ruptured ovarian cyst . . . *You wouldn't even bother* doing a physical examination looking for the ovarian cyst . . ." (page 360-361). "I can't think of anything you would find on the second day [during pelvic exam] . . ." (page 362). "You wouldn't do a pelvic the second day looking for ovarian cysts . . ." (also page 362). But, expert, having access to the summary of the complete exam one month ago would help us focus away from the possibility of PID (which I had swabbed for) and ectopic pregnancy given that her last sexual partner had been more than a year previously; but in a woman who had had her last period four months ago and whom I had examined one month ago, there *could still be* an (1) ovarian cyst, (2) periovarian tenderness from a recent cyst rupture, (3) ovulation pain, (4) an ovarian cyst torsion, or (5) a recent bleed into the wall of an ovarian cyst rendering it hemorrhagic. All are reasonable causes of abdominal pain in a woman who has this presentation, but definitely not the presentation of an appendicitis or PID. And if there is a chain of three to four centimeter pellets of firm stool in a redundant sigmoid colon in the pelvic vicinity, a diligent examiner will want to empty the bowel to be sure that he/she is examining the actual ovaries, in a nonurgent situation such as this was. See what I wrote in chapter 1 about a similar situation. Ironic that the situations are so similar, isn't it? And did I proceed in an identical fashion? You bet I did! Identical!

"Both a rectal and a pelvic exam are no more uncomfortable than just one of them" (page 349). Ouch! I dare say, virtually every single female reader of this book will disagree, Ms. Expert. Why even say such a dumb thing? But you are a woman on a mission, aren't you?

She says, "I can't comment what most family physicians do . . ." (page 350). But isn't that the whole point of the hearing – to determine whether a physician has performed his duties consistent with the standard among his peers? Compare this to college council's totally uninformed assertion (page 264) – that Dr. Expert shows the exact standard that Dr. Litchfield should be held to. This was the exchange in the hearing as to whether she should be considered qualified as an expert witness:

My lawyer: "Well, my position is this: I agree that Dr Expert is qualified to give expert opinion in these areas. The question is to how much weight should be given to her opinion as someone who is not in primary practice – in primary care in family practice, is going to be an issue for the committee at the end of the day, but I agree she can give the evidence. The point being, that she is not, in any sense, Dr Litchfield's peer. She has a different field of practice."

Mr. BBBB: "And my simple response to that is Dr Expert has already spoken to that she actually teaches students, including family residents, who are the peers of Dr Litchfield, so it speaks to the very issue of what is the appropriate standard that is taught to family residents, family physicians, so my friend and I can argue about what weight, but I would say that she can provide expert opinion evidence which is directly on point to what is the standard that we are dealing with provided in relation to Dr Litchfield's practice." [I agree, his grammar here is awful.]

So then, all family doctors should practice medicine the way referral surgeons do? Is *this quackery* an official college policy? Is it going to be a bylaw?

INSISTENCE ON RECTAL EXAM

Mme L'Expert impresses us by saying, "Well, he could find out pretty quickly by putting his finger in the rectum: liquid VS solid stool VS empty rectum" (page 355). "If he's so thorough, then why didn't he do that [a rectal exam]?" (page 356). While I could have done it, *I didn't need to do a rectal exam* for stool on this patient because I had already felt large pelletlike stool lumps in her redundant sigmoid colon and rectum when I did the preliminary vaginal exam the first day. So to use your own words of accusation, such a *rectal exam would, then, have been "unnecessary" and, therefore, inappropriate! Wouldn't that make any physician who did both when the first made the second unnecessary, guilty of conduct unbecoming a physician?* Does the college expert propose the need to check for a retrorectal appendicitis? Certainly a retrocecal appendicitis we have all heard of; was she proposing that one might occur retrorectally?

I knew this wasn't the presentation of the infection state that accompanies appendicitis or pelvic inflammatory disease, so I didn't need to do a rectal exam or a white blood count in this patient, but I didn't have the final diagnosis for her on that first day. The second pelvic exam, the next day, allowed me to confirm that with the laxative measures she had emptied the sigmoid colon of those lumps *and* discern any lumps actually associated with the ovaries. That is what I did – I excluded ovarian pathology.

And Dr. L'Expert makes *specific exception of the ovaries*: "You can feel those same organs, *minus the ovaries*, through the rectal" (page 356). So she actually *says* "minus the ovaries." In this expert's opinion, then, the ovaries are not important in the assessment of a woman's abdominal pain? She, of course, doesn't actually believe this but didn't want to agree with my lawyer because she thought that if she did, she might lose *HER case*! Her case? But wait! Isn't that *contrary to the role* of an expert witness? And all this time, the assistant registrar is watching/observing and not attempting to remind her of her role in the hearing. (What's that about, sir? Did we not used to be colleagues? Have I offended you in some *previous lifetime?*)

Then she sort of meanders. "PID is frequently missed because they don't do a pelvic exam looking for vaginal discharge" (page 366). Then you're saying that doctors don't always look for a discharge and so miss pelvic inflammatory disease?" But (page 283) now wait! By the same reasoning that we applied to nipple discharge – if the patient doesn't complain of it, then it isn't there, right? So if the patient doesn't complain of vaginal discharge, PID is not there, right? At least that would be consistent, in a quirky way. Do you feel comfortable with that, Ms. Expert? Reader, is that the way you want your doctor to practice? In regard to this issue, I had in fact obtained a history one month before, including date of last intercourse being more than a year previously, and no vaginal discharge of significance. And my notes from that exam were face up in the chart on the page just previous – easily available for reference. Also, from that exam one month before, *I had done a cervical swab*, so if there was any PID (an infection from a previous partner) present then, it would have shown up on the lab results. There just was none! Of the many causes of abdominal pain, given the history of no regular menstruation and no intercourse, *ovarian examination was, actually, Expert, very, very important* on the ninth and, when uncertain, the tenth of August (the next day after evacuating the bowel)!

WHAT DID THE COMMITTEE INFER THIS TIME?

What did the committee find? Page 18: they found that Dr. Expert should declare what my findings were! "She stated that his findings on the first visit were that of *constipation only* [Golly! It must have been difficult for the panel to agree to that since the chart itself says otherwise. This committee has clearly allowed itself to *deny the presence* of what they can actually read!] and, when resolved by his treatment to the patient's satisfaction, [in clear contradiction to what both the chart and I said – still pain and tenderness the second day] that a vaginal re-examination was unnecessary."

Further, *they allowed that they, too, could replace what my findings were*: "He appeared to suggest that with hard pellets behind the back wall of the vagina on vaginal exam, that constipation was the *only* feature in his impression that day." But my chart clearly says that there was *abdominal pain AND constipation*. And that some abdominal pain and tenderness were still there the next day! By *permitting themselves* to deny the very words that the chart held, they declared, "A repeat vaginal exam is found to be inappropriate on day two and therefore allegation 14 is proven and the defendant is found guilty. His actions strongly suggest *motives that are focused on the examination of a patient's vaginal area*, to the exclusion of what a caring physician would have done. His actions are, therefore, unbecoming of a Physician." What do you think, committee? Was this contrivance your proudest moment? Or, were your own actions unbecoming of a two physicians and a social worker?

MANUAL THERAPY DIFFERENCES

The osteopath is brought to say that to examine the paraspinous soft tissue does not require anterior chest counterpressure . . . it is unnecessary and therefore wrong! (But what he is actually saying is, "It is *unnecessary for Me* to apply anterior chest counter-pressure *because I do the exam with the patient lying face-down on a table or bed*, and . . . the table . . . is providing the counter pressure.") Oh, that's why you say it is *unnecessary* to provide anterior counterpressure when doing a standing or sitting thoracic spine exam because you don't do it standing or sitting? Unnecessary doesn't necessarily equal inappropriate, does it?

Expert Witness 2, you say that you don't ever do an upright examination of the thoracic spine. You only do it with the patient prone. Of course, with that technique you would never need any counterpressure on the front of the body because the examining bench or table would provide the counterpressure. So Litchfield must be a pervert. I get it. Shucks, and I didn't think I was. Well, you've convinced me. I must be a pervert for doing an upright exam of the thoracic spine. OK! I guess I might as well take my lumps.

But . . . could you just answer one more question? Do ALL doctors of osteopathy do things the way you say that you do? *Are you sure you know?* If you are saying that I should be found guilty of inappropriate exams, don't you need to be kind of sure?

Is it not possible that Dr. R Todd Dombroski (director, Madigan Army Medical Center, Sports Medicine Clinic, Tacoma, Washington); Dr. Harry D. Friedman (assistant professor, San Francisco College of Osteopathic Medicine and Michigan State University College of Osteopathic Medicine); and Michael A Seffinger (instructor, Osteopathic Medicine, Pacific Hospital of Long Beach Family Practice Residency Program), all doctors of esteopathy, emphasized to me the appropriateness of upright thoracic spine exams on 9 September 1995 at the AAFP Scientific Assembly in Anaheim? Those of us who do this exam upright know that if the body is not trapped between a front-restraining and back-palpating hand, it will either *tip forward* OR the patient will push back in order to resist the slight-yet-real pressure from behind. And this tightening of the thoracic paraspinous extensor muscles will do what, sir? Come on, you know the answer. *It will compromise the very tissue that we are trying to assess* by gentle palpation! And we both know that when we are palpating for somatic dysfunction, it's not like feeling for a bone out of place or a firm true muscle spasm. And we both know that when we provide an appropriate intervention and then recheck, that subtle difference in tissue tone that you and I call somatic dysfunction will have disappeared immediately!

However, we also know that the technique that I employ in reducing somatic dysfunction in the upright thorax is a thrust-type maneuver. Provider beware! *We don't do it* on patients with thoracic osseous malignancy (bone cancer in the rib cage), rheumatoid arthritis, previous sternotomy (as in cardiac bypass surgery), Down's Syndrome, an acute rib fracture, severe osteoporosis, or costochondritis. Why is that, sir? Come on, you know the answer. It's because *we can make them worse*! That's right! When you know 'em just call 'em out! In fairness to Dr. Expert 2, he does say (page 381), in answer to the ultimately unfair and imbalanced question about inadvertent contact with the breast by Mr. BBBB, "Would, in your description of incidental contact, that include – and this is dealing with a back exam – one hand from behind *cupping* a breast?" [Mr. BBBB wants this phrase – *cupping a breast* – to be used over and over so that it might seem that that actually happened.] Now Dr. Expert 2 doesn't even grace that goofy question with a direct answer, but instead says, "In my experience, the – and the teachings from the osteopathic background, that should not be necessary for examination of the thoracic spine or the upper back, although there may be need for anterior contact *if the chest wall structures themselves needed to be examined*." So he is acting like a real expert witness and would understand how an examining doctor might want to exclude acute inflammatory processes and fractures. The college lawyer wants to limit that evidence, though.

Remember, Dr. Expert 2, I didn't do these things right from my medical school days like you did. I learned them over time and added them gradually to my approach, from almost ten years after my graduation. But I did learn in medical school what a chest compression test for rib fracture was. And when I started doing manual medicine, I wanted to be darned sure I would not cause harm with a thrust maneuver because so many in the medical profession criticized the chiropractic profession, which we basically didn't know much about – for all its "dangerous manipulations." I achieved awareness of fractures and inflammation by putting one hand directly on the skin overlying the sternum, and the other palpating paraspinously with a little bit of anterior pressure over those costosternal junctures to rule out sternochondritis. It can also disclose a barely symptomatic rib fracture.

AND THE COMMITTEE FIGURED?

Now then, the committee wanted to get its own two cents in as they pressed me along the road to the gallows. The committee took Dr. Expert 2's testimony to mean "that there should be *no need* for anterior contact with the patient's chest to stabilize for torque when simply palpating lightly for tissue tone, but might be necessary when performing resistance type range of motion testing." But they failed to understand that college expert 2 does his palpation with the *patient LYING FACEDOWN!* So really the table or examining bench provides that anterior counterpressure, doesn't it, committee?

The committee also chose *the most assaultive view* of checking the pectoralis muscle for tightness when the opposing trapezius and medial-to-scapula muscles were tight in a woman who'd said she had a frozen shoulder. Much of the pectoral muscle does lie behind the breast, and their view was that there must have been a lot of *breast fondling* and hence, sexual boundary crossing in its examination. They didn't have to ask me whether during that assessment my hand would have made contact with the breast because fondling fit the bias that they were forming. The way I actually do it is to palpate just the myotendinous area where real shortening and tenderness can be discovered. For those of you not medical, that means to feel the anterior axillary fold – the front boundary of *the armpit!* Well, it's not as spicy as fondling a breast, of course, but a trained physician can learn a lot that way.

Remember, in this lady, the range of neck motion was reduced in all directions. As a little personal experiment on this issue, hold your elbow in a fixed position to your front lateral (side) chest wall and look as high as you can overhead. Pick a spot on the ceiling – maybe, climb up there and put a little mark on the ceiling. So when you look overhead with your shoulder frozen, that's how far you can see, right? Now "unfreeze" your shoulder and bring your shoulder blades together behind you and look up overhead again. You should get at least seven to ten degrees more. You can see farther? Good, you've understood. True frozen shoulder can limit your range of neck extension. And that issue would be what I was checking for with the palpation of the *not-so-sexy* front of the armpit.

The committee goes on to say (findings, page 7), "The credibility of Dr Litchfield's actions gave the panel *grave concerns.* We could find no credible reason that his hand placed against her bare skin, hidden from his view [remember that I had resolved to keep patients as dressed in their own clothing as they could be kept – leaving them in as many of their own things as possible because of my previous criticisms from the College] and underneath her shirt could have any clinical or diagnostic purpose. *His assertion* that he was attempting to check for costochondral tenderness (costochondritis) *is not believable* given that the costochondral junctions are not even at the sternal border where he states his hand was purposefully placed. *Even more sinister* was the fact that his efforts were designed to place his hand on the patient's bare skin instead of over her clothes, for instance." Wow! There you've got me! I called inflammation of the chondrosternal junctions chostochondritis! Eee gads! I'm awful! *I must really be a pervert!* I should just go quietly to the gallows, right?

But then, I thought, *That IS, what I call costochondritis!*

So was the committee right? Am I guilty of conduct unbecoming a physician for calling swelling and tenderness right where the sternum meets the cartilaginous portions of the ribs, costochondritis? It's a little hard to imagine, but what do other physicians around here call it? And here is where I applied my research background and Dr. Expert 1's "if you ask 100 physicians" phrase.

AND THE SURVEY SAYS

I figured I would prepare a black-and-white copy of figure 5-13 of my copy of the *Atlas of Clinical Anatomy* by Richard S Snell published in 1978 by Little Brown and Company Inc. I then took that photocopy of the thorax and circled the fourth, fifth, and sixth chondrosternal junctures and took it to forty physicians whom I knew from the Royal Alexandra Hospital where I did family practice rounds, the University of Alberta Hospital where I had surgical assisting privileges, extended care doctors with Capital Care and Good Samaritan Hospitals where I had staff meetings, and the Edmonton Doctor's Curling League where I played for four years against teams sometimes skipped by none other than the registrar (and he is very, very competitive)! I asked each of these forty colleagues [but not him] while pointing to my circled junctures, "If you found swelling, inflammation, and tenderness here, here, and here, what is that called?"

This was rather a fun project for me, and I really looked for some fun in the midst of the "storm of outrageous oppression." I ended up talking with an emergency room doctor, an ophthalmologist, fourteen family physicians, one thoracic surgeon, eight orthopedic surgeons, six anesthesiologists, a pulmonologist (lung doctor), a rehabilitation doctor, a pathologist, a cardiologist, a hematologist, a general and pediatric surgeon, an endocrinologist, an internist, and finally one rheumatologist who had previously been a member of the council. Two gave me very good anatomically descriptive names; one said there was no diagnosis, and one would not give me an answer. *The other thirty-six agreed with me that this was called costochondritis!* The last one I saw was the rheumatologist. I actually made an appointment to ask him my question. Because he had recently served on the Council of the College, I was nervous. Even though I had gathered all the other answers by then, I really wanted his affirmation (because he was a specialist in joint disorders) . . . and he gave it! As best I can recall, he said, "Well, of course, Bryant, *we all call this costochondritis.* But I'm not convinced that it is a real disease by itself . . . and any interventions to treat it should really be quite innocuous." He agreed with me as to its name – that is the point! I loved his accent and his handlebar mustache – just between you and me!

So is my assertion that I was ruling out costochondritis *unbelievable?* Certainly, if I am sinister for this, there are these other thirty-six out of forty Edmonton physicians (90%) who are equally sinister. Should we all be erased from the registry? *Whose registry is it, anyway?* Or, is it becoming a private club?

The evidence had shown that with a chaperone present (in an effort to enable the patient to keep *wearing as much of her own clothing* as possible due to my second conclusion after the prior complaints) when a bra strap was in my way, I asked permission to undo it, and then did so if verbal permission was given. The biased committee criticized me repeatedly for this during the hearing. They could not let the appropriate descriptive phrase: "unclasping or undoing" the bra strap stand but referred to it as "removing the bra." Why would they do that? Of course, to make it *sound* worse! In any case, I arranged to go to the only boundaries course for physicians in Canada – it is in Ontario, put on by the University of Western Ontario for the College of Physicians and Surgeons of Ontario. Part of the course involved our examination of professional patients (who had been given a script to go by) while the other physicians and the MD course directors watched to provide later comment. I did this on the eighth and ninth of April 2005. Can you guess which script my patient had been given? Yup! She was told to be someone with chest pain and a cough and wasn't to be willing to remove her clothing or let me undo her bra! I did ask permission, which she denied me. So in the end, I did the best exam I could do under those circumstances. Those who critiqued me gave me full marks for asking, for respecting her right to decline, and for proceeding in the way I best could. In the course syllabus there is a checklist that REQUIRES that one specifically *ask permission to open a bra, and then proceed to do so.* The asking and the opening were *mandatory* for this course specifically on doctor-patient boundaries. This course on boundary violations did not consider that to be one, committee. They upheld my use of this practice!

DOING A PELVIC EXAM TO UNDERSTAND MECHANICS

From page 384: Expert 2 had also written in his response to the college's seeking his opinion: "From the information that was provided, it appeared that there was *frequent use* of internal vaginal examinations in the evaluation of low back pain . . ." That must imply wrongfulness, right? So why on earth would a fella trained like me do a vaginal exam in a situation like this? This was a woman who had incurred a traumatic broken tailbone seven weeks before. What is a broken tailbone? Wow . . . well, it's . . . a fracture . . . or break . . . of a tailbone . . . you know . . . that place where our tail comes from, right?

How are you feeling about this? Enlightened? No, nor I. The word *tailbone* is ambiguous and therefore not medically useful. Let's add just a touch of science to this confusion. Is a "broken tailbone"

1. a posttraumatic coccydynia (bruised coccyx)?
2. a true fracture of the sacrum?
3. a dislocation of the little chain of seven coccygeal bones, that is *"all or some of the seven" still anteriorly dislocated* seven weeks

later (when she came to the rural emergency room where I was working) and healing in that crooked fashion?

And furthermore, did items 1-3 above have anything to do with her presenting complaint of pain running down the leg, sciatica-like? If so, is there anything that we could do about it? Well, my purpose is to actually clarify things for you.

1. A posttraumatic coccydynia is a bruised coccyx. It can continue to be a source of pain for months or years after injury, but the pain is usually localized right to the bruise site. When it becomes chronic, it is because we keep sitting on it. Traumatic coccydynia can be improved by long-acting local anaesthetic injections (sometimes with steroid) and donut cushions.
2. An undisplaced fracture of the sacrum would likely be healed by seven weeks. A displaced sacral fracture would usually be associated with other pelvic fractures. Patients usually can't walk when this happens.
3. An anterior dislocation of the lower three to seven coccygeal bones could certainly be present. These little bones are almost always too small to break, but somewhere in the chain, they can dislocate forward. Can you guess how that is checked (even seven weeks later, at one in the morning in a rural hospital where x-ray would have to be called in)? Did you say a vaginal or rectal exam to look for the forward bend in that chain of bones? That's right! Good job! You understand your anatomy!

What else could possibly cause pressure on the nerves going to the leg? Just a hint, this is a middle-aged woman. Think through a listing of pathologic etiology. Is it inherited from birth or acquired? The history says it's acquired – she didn't used to have it. What are its origins? Toxic? Unlikely. Vascular? Unlikely. Metabolic? Unlikely. Infectious/inflammatory? Possibly – like an abscess? Good thinking. Neoplastic? Yes, cancer can occur at any age. In this woman, there could be an ovarian tumor. Degenerative? Unlikely. Traumatic? We have discussed above. Oh, by the way, do you guys even watch *House*?

My own literature search to find the tender trigger point proximal to the ischial spine mentioned in *The Team Physician's Handbook* printed in 1990 was more profitable than the "almost negligible" literature search done by Dr. Expert 1. It led me to an article by Durrani and Winnie titled "Piriformis Muscle Syndrome: An Underdiagnosed Cause of Sciatica" published in the *Journal of Pain and Symptom Management* Vol. 6, No. 6, in August 1991. In their table 4 is listed the "Frequency of Positive Physical Signs." Let's go through them:

1. Rectal/pelvic exam – 26/26=100%
2. Deep digital palpation of piriformis muscle – 24/26=92.3%
3. Sacroiliac tenderness – 10/26=38.5%
4. Pace's Sign – 8/26=30.8%
5. Freiberg's sign – 9/26=34.6%
6. Lasegue's sign – 12/26=46.2%
7. Piriformis sign – 10/26=38.5%

Now I know that the vast majority of you are NOT doctors, but I think you can draw conclusions from this obvious information pretty well. Much of medicine is taught (painfully) by questioning. So here's the big question, which of the physical signs ALWAYS confirms piriformis syndrome? (I'll give you one hint; it has the 100 percent beside it.) Yes, that's right! Rectal or vaginal exam! You got it right again! In fairness, deep external palpation of the piriformis muscle also has a high frequency of positivity, but it lacks a LOT of *specificity* (that means it doesn't specify which muscle the pain is coming from!). The tenderness that is felt by palpating the buttock can certainly come from the much larger gluteus maximus, which overlies the much deeper piriformis muscle.

The committee in its findings stated that "the articles presented on this topic agreed in that there might well be tenderness elicited on deep pelvic exam in pyriformis [same as piriformis] syndrome, but that external methods *are just as good if not better.*" Wow! Now I feel guilty!

But . . . wait, "just as good [as rectal/pelvic exam] if not better"? Are any of the methods just as good as 100 percent? And then, *is it possible to be better than 100 percent?* But wait, it just gets better! Remember, too, that it says pelvic OR rectal exam. The committee then says, "The most critical fact with regard to the performance of a vaginal exam in this instance was that Dr Litchfield was attempting to assess the pubococcygeus muscles which border the vaginal walls. They *have nothing to do* with the pyriformis muscles at the back of the pelvis." Well, committee doctors, at least *YOU* don't know of any association between the pubococcygeus and the piriformis. I do believe that. Probably the social worker doesn't either, but I'm just guessing here, perhaps she does. However, a link between those two muscles has actually been known in medicine for a long, long time. Reference to this fact is present in the Winnie and Durrani bibliography at the back of their article. Reference 16: Thiele GH. "Tonic spasm of levator ani, coccygeus, and piriformis muscle." Trans Am Pract Soc 1936; 37: 145-155. You see my friends, the tightening happens at the same time, so the most easily accessible muscle, the (pubo)coccygeus, can also provide information on the harder to reach piriformis muscle. This is an example of muscle recruitment – muscles *near* an injured muscle also tighten up, as everyone who has had a car accident can attest to on the second day. Notice the date of that article – way back in 1936. I trust that this was not taught in the medical schools that the doctors on the committee went to. Hence, their suppositions.

So let's summarize the reasons to do a pelvic exam on the lady in question:

1. To rule out persistent *dislocation* of some of the coccygeal bones in a woman who says she had a "broken tailbone" seven weeks before (remember, we CAN fix a dislocation).
2. To be sure that there is no huge pelvic/ovarian *abscess or tumor.*
3. To determine if the *pubococcygeus* (and by inference, the piriformis) muscle had obvious increased tone on one side of the pelvis.

So then, what is Dr. Expert 2's approach to this issue. If a pelvic exam could give us a lot more information about a big problem for such a patient, what do you do, Expert 2? Come on, everyone wants to know! *And his answer is, "I refer it away* [to a female pelvic floor physiotherapist]!" So when you say that pelvic exam for piriformis syndrome is unnecessary, nay inappropriate it is because *you would have it done by someone else?* That is your answer? Oh my goodness! Really? Now is *THAT* an official policy of the college? By that crazy policy (watch out, it may become a bylaw), *ALL EXAMS* could be construed as unnecessary/inappropriate because they could all be *done by someone else*, don't cha' know (page 385 and 386 of the transcripts)!

Doctor Expert 2's office reports that although he does pelvic exams and Pap smears for his family practice patients, "he likes to keep osteopathy separate from his family practice." So if a need for pelvic floor assessment were present, it would not be by him, but by someone he referred the patient to. Well, at least this helps make health care less expensive . . . NOT! This approach would not be appropriate for me. My copy of the *Team Physician's Handbook* by Mellion, Walsh, and Shelton published by Hanley & Belfus, Inc in 1990 defined piriformis syndrome as an "irritation of the sciatic nerve as it passes underneath or through the piriformis muscle producing a deep localized pain in the posterior aspect of the hip [near the sciatic notch] that often radiates down into the leg." It added that "a history of trauma can only be elicited in approximately half the cases, and the nature of the trauma is seldom dramatic." Page 398 further adds that there may be a history of pain on intercourse in females and that it occurs "about six times more frequently in women than in men." This excellent textbook goes on to explain three other important things:

1. "Both active external rotation of the hip against resistance, and passive stretch into internal rotation will produce pain [on the affected side]."
2. "On pelvic and/or rectal exam, there is often a *distinct*, tender, trigger point proximal to the ischial spine; during palpation

the patient will experience pain and often exclaim that this is the first time someone has found 'my pain.'"

3. "*It is difficult to diagnose with any certainty* and may be a diagnosis of exclusion."

Well now, I got this book shortly after it was produced in 1990. Remember, after those initial complaints in 1989, I had resolved to learn a better and more thorough approach to back exam. But what was the exact anatomic location of the "tender trigger point proximal to [beside] the ischial spine"? Beside the ischial spine, there are three significant muscles that together form the levator ani (the anus lifter) and therefore, the pelvic floor. They are the pubococcygeus, the iliococcygeus, and the coccygeus muscles. And that's what these muscles have to do with the piriformis muscle, gang! Your "committee" certainly had no clue.

DANGER OF COMMITTEE USING ITS OWN EVIDENCE

In their total ignorance, but with bias that I had already been found (in their limited view) guilty of crossing over sexual boundaries on other things, they stated, "The articles presented on this topic agreed that there might well be tenderness elicited on deep pelvic exam in piriformis syndrome, but that external methods are *just as good if not better*. The panel believes that the appropriateness of a vaginal exam in practice is *vastly* different to the circumstances in an investigational study."

"The most CRITICAL fact with regard to the performance of a vaginal exam in this instance was that Dr Litchfield was attempting to assess the pubococcygeus muscles which border the vaginal walls. They have nothing to do with the pyriformis muscles at the back of the pelvis. He did not demonstrate any *attempt to relax the patient* and attempt a deep pelvic exam to determine if there was any tenderness at the back wall of the pelvis." Now here we need to cite some true but unpleasant further science. In a woman who has had three babies and then goes on to middle age, the vaginal introitus (opening) and support muscles are very slack. One of my dear young moms who'd only had one baby (but before marriage) asked me several years later to arrange for her "that surgery that makes you a virgin again." [I wonder if that, too, is popular in California.] I mourn for the young women of our day who are swept by this kind of fad and are made to feel less than adequate without it.

After having babies, there is a lot of associated bladder incontinence as middle age is achieved. Bladder repairs and attempts to lessen the descent of pelvic organs are common in the middle age group of women. The very purpose of having an AP (anterior and posterior) repair is to deal with this *common laxity*. The idea of attempting to relax the vaginal opening in this group of women would only be suggested by those ignorant of this fact. But remember the article that you just read talked of this evidence being confirmatory by EITHER vaginal OR rectal exam. Is the committee suggesting that the article recommends palpating the piriformis muscle directly VIA THE RECTUM? I urgently suggest you don't consider trying to reach the piriformis muscle *by rectal* exam: you would cause permanent damage even with your supposed efforts "to relax the patient"! When you don't know a subject, don't assume that you can guess pretty well because of your "training."

Only with not-so-deep gloved hand exam through the vagina: (1) each now-very-small or not-at-all palpable ovary was noted, (2) the tip of the coccyx was checked for its position and alignment, and (3) each pubococcygeus muscle was palpated. Only these facts were important; no attempt was made to reach the piriformis muscle pelvically or rectally. Did the committee interpret the Durrani article to infer that the examiner reached the piriformis muscle via rectal exam? Think for a moment: you are virtually certain to rupture the anal sphincter trying that!

Of the vaginal exam that this patient certainly *did* anticipate, the committee said, "He simply invaded the patient's privacy without warning, explanation or consent *when no diagnostic benefit* was to be gained. The doctor's grossly apparent lack of attention to the invasions of her privacy without any form of explanation or consent proves a conduct that *shows no concern* for the patient's well being, and therefore unbecoming conduct for a Physician . . . The panel has determined that there is an overwhelming balance of probability that the vaginal exam in this instance was inappropriate, had no clinical merit and was *a gross invasion* of the patient's privacy. He is therefore found guilty of unbecoming conduct in a professional capacity."

Wow! That is damning! *Did you say "an Overwhelming Balance of probability"?* I must just be no good at all. Or else this committee's guesses may be totally erroneous! The members of the committee suggest, it would seem, that the only way to examine the very deep piriformis muscle internally would be to deeply relax the patient in question, and then go at it from the vagina OR the RECTUM. Let me again discourage you from EVER attempting to reach the piriformis muscle from the rectum of even a very, very relaxed patient: you will rupture the anal sphincter and need to refer the patient for repair! A patient treated this way might well make a complaint to the college, and then a hearing committee might be asking you questions and stressing your life. This is one of the reasons it is bad form to intermittently interject your own "deep medical knowledge" into a hearing about issues you are not especially savvy to. This, in your official capacity as judges, makes the hearing more unfair, of course.

CHAPTER 5

COMPLAINANTS: THE FINAL FOUR

WHY DOES A PATIENT MAKE A COMPLAINT?

There are probably five main reasons:

1. They really were assaulted. I must sadly admit that I know at least three doctors who did this.
2. They want to assist a friend who claims that she was assaulted – to add weight to the likelihood of her claim.
3. They had an exam with which they were uncomfortable/ not familiar, and another doctor, their psychologist, an older woman, or a *trusted friend said* that it was not appropriate. Can you see how easily this can proceed? It just may mean that the second physician/other person was *not aware* of the technique? Like the registrar, the expert, and the committee in this case. However, a cascade of further accusations can ensue.
4. They are litigious. That means they like to sue people in socially vulnerable positions, to make money. This is, of course, fraud.

But some college personnel may actually believe the tale or use the complainant to achieve *their own* ends.

5. They feel guilty. Now you weren't expecting that one, were you? Well, there are two possibilities:
   - Guilt for having some quasi-sexual feelings.
   - Guilt for allowing something to be done to her that she had been told was sexual.

Clearly, some explanation is in order. I am the father of five boys and four girls. My wife and I spent long hours teaching our girls where not to allow boys to touch them, and our boys (albeit, less frequently) were not to touch girls. I am very aware that in the course of my annual attendance on the average female in my practice, between age 18 and 106, I touch them in all of the warned-of places. Now, if guilt does arise, they can either feel guilty that they have allowed my touching, *OR* it is remotely possible (but not very predictable) that they actually felt some sexual pleasure at being touched. This puts male physicians more in the "line of fire" than their female counterparts. Or it did, until statistics showed that the same percentage of lesbian representation in the general population was present among female physicians. Now the aware – but insecure – have no haven in seeking a female physician. Theoretically, either sex could have an interest in them sexually.

This last issue – feeling guilty about what they allowed a boy or man to do TO them – has other ramifications. Some young women, then, grow up believing that their sexuality is what they allow to be done TO them. Some of them don't ever get past that. That would mean they don't become active in their own sexuality – they remain completely passive. They let certain boys or men do this or that to them. They are really a sexual object. Now that sounds more like the Hugh Hefner definition. And he can really sell it. Imagine, an industry selling back to you your own sexuality! Very beautiful women may actually come away from that mistaken premise believing that they are so amazing that all they have to do is allow things to be done to them! Be passive. Let the guys do all the initiating. As a woman, you aren't really a person – you are an object! To be acted upon. Do you feel comfortable with that? I sure don't! Other than the five reasons that I have given, can you think of any other reasons to claim inappropriate behavior from a physician?

1. JM:

This lady was a friend of PV. They had both come to Edmonton, from the Maritimes. They both had emotional baggage that they brought with them. I saw them both early in 2001. They both needed help. Where PV had been abandoned by each of the four men who had impregnated her, JM was single and anxious. She didn't trust herself. She didn't trust her choices. She did not think she was worth much. Through a local psychologist, each lady ended up seeing me for their medical, prescription, and some additional counseling needs. As a part of my care, I did a complete medical on each of them. They were the closest of friends. At times, they each irritated the heck out of the other. Being an unsure adult is fraught with challenges. You can't trust anyone . . . because you can't trust yourself! And you've got years of history to prove it. PV had two children by men who left her. She had also had two abortions – I suspect during two previous pregnancies from equally uncaring men. Four for four! This lady had learned to be rejected. What a difficult path. The rejections sensitize a girl to the early signs of rejection. She was very experienced at being rejected and shared her life experiences with JM. I *cared for them each*, and I cared *about* them each. I could see how life's sculpting had made them the way they were. They were a part of the same religious faith that I held. I was no better than they, but I did have a loving wife and nine healthy children. My home was a happy home.

JM was trying to become educated and then employed. I think she was just under thirty years old. She often tended PV's kids when needed. PV was not employed. Maybe she was just in survival mode. Maybe PV took advantage of JM a bit. The latter did complain to me of that. A person only has five possible types of emotional supports: spouse, family, friends, work, and religion.

1. Neither was working.
2. Family was in the Maritimes.
3. Neither had a spouse.
4. Each had few friends apart from each other.

Neither was very supported according to these criteria. But they did share my religion. And it can be very, very supportive!

After JM had been my patient for a time, she booked a complete medical. This is a good idea for every new patient. The day she came for the medical, I took her history in my usual very organized way. There was a family history of mental illness and breast cancer, but JM herself never did breast self-exams. She had also just started her period. In the course of the physical exam, I spent time teaching her breast self-examination. When I do this, I do a clinical breast exam including an attempt to express ductal secretions. Then I put the patient's hand under my hand and enable her to feel what I have felt. I do not teach patients to express secretions unless they are about to begin breast-feeding, but the rest of my clinical breast exam I teach them (with tactile experience) to do on themselves. Then we go to the other side and repeat – first me and then the patient. The other side should be a mirror image of the first. One of them said of this that she'd understood with my teaching on one side, so why on earth did I do the other side with her? What she doesn't know is that as a part of my continuing medical education, I was taught with one hundred models of breasts and ten women with abnormalities. Sadly, one time through doesn't make you an expert, PV.

Breast sizes may not be identical, but the configuration should be. That means, if there is a prominence on one side there should be a symmetrical prominence on the other side. The order of my sequence in physical exam puts the breast exam after the supine cardiac exam. Then I examine the abdomen and, subsequently, do the pelvic exam. However, JM had started her period that day, so we deferred that. The palpation portion of the pelvic could have been done during menstruation, but the speculum exam and Pap smear at that time would be of little value since the cervical cells scraped from the cervix would be less well seen under the microscope in the presence of considerable blood cells. So we decided that she would rebook the entire pelvic exam.

She returned for the pelvic at a time when she was no longer menstruating. There were *findings that day* that were *inconsistent* with what the patient had told me of her history. It was awkward for me – she had a completely intact hymen, despite having said that she had had intercourse previously. And she had said that she was able to orgasm. This latter is certainly possible without penetration, so her account might have been completely accurate in that regard. However, I had to use a pediatric metal speculum to do the Pap smear and the swab on her because her hymen resisted anything beyond the first portion of my gloved index finger. I told her, "Wow, JM, this is great! [Because of our shared faith] I don't know exactly what you did in your sexual encounters, but you are medically still a virgin!" I have heard that some fellows have a very narrow erect penis, but the only size that could have penetrated her would have been about a seven – to ten-year-old child. I have never seen an adult male with that size penis. I thought I was the bringer of good news to her – she was still a virgin, technically! I think the news was not so good to her, though. She had gotten used to believing that she was an experienced, used, woman of the world, and here I was telling her the contrary. This may have made her feel, again, unsure of herself. My information may somehow have contributed further to her already negative perception of herself.

Months later, in the course of counseling when she had secured an HR (human resources management – the area of her studies) job, she departed from our theme that day to ask me why, when I had examined her breasts those months ago, I had attempted to express the ducts. She may have referred to this as squeezing the nipples, but that would be a very lay interpretation of the technique. I did not have a copy of the original 1976 DeGowin and DeGowin *Textbook of Physical Exam* at that time in my office, but I had Don Novey's 1990 *Rapid Access Guide to the Physical Examination* right on my shelf in the next room. It showed with photographs the exact technique that I had learned textually from the DeGowin and DeGowin book. I wanted to reassure her that proper technique had been observed. I recalled Burt Lancestor's supporting role in Kevin Costner's *Field of Dreams*. He plays an old-time country doctor who tells Kevin, who has somehow found him from the past, that he'd "best be gettin' home to the wife" 'cause he wouldn't want her to be thinkin' he'd found a mistress. In what I could muster of that dear old actor's spirit, I expressed that "I would not want you [her] to get to thinkin' that your [her] doctor was coming onto you [her]!" She seemed to be satisfied by my explanation at that time.

I think she got a job at a women's shelter with her new HR qualifications. I can imagine that she had to fill out some paperwork for the job. I can imagine what they would have told her when she informed them of the name of her new family physician: Dr. Bryant Litchfield. I suspect that the media hype that had *publicly fizzled out* from my previous trials was still alive and well at the sexual assault center and some of the women's shelters. What did her new job administration tell her that they "knew" about me? Or, did she talk with another physician who didn't do the exam the way I had? Or, did she talk to the psychologist who had referred her to me, and that woman had not been examined the way that I was using? Or did she talk with a nursing student, medical student, older female friend, cab driver, florist, airline pilot, part-time clown, or pastry chef. Now here, I hope you see some of the humor that I intended. Maybe something inside you says that I should not find humor in this serious business. You know what? I think I've *earned the right* to use humor to find what comfort I can. Check out my chapter on how these proceedings have hurt me. But I must also tell you that this person with no personal assurance, no self-esteem – a person who doubts herself, may feel just as able to trust one as any other of these "random acquaintances." Not because each of them is doubtful, but because she doubts herself.

For whichever of these or other reasons, she later became uncertain of the answer I had given her, and hence . . . of me! Had she again chosen poorly in creating and building with me a professional relationship? The thought must have been painful to her, leaving her another in the continual hurts from males in her life. Did she inform the psychologist who sent her to me that she felt betrayed by that lady for exposing her to a previously publicly denounced pervert?

Did the psychologist feel, with the new information, that she might be right? Was there forever to be an awkward distance between that psychologist and I?

JM's complaint to the college was made in honesty. I reviewed my training with assistant registrar for the college. He understood that I was correctly following my medical training, as you now also understand. But the "small dog" had to report to the "BIG DOG," who was, then, the chairman of the complaints committee. Something got "lost in translation." This chairman may not have been aware of the teaching of breast exam the way I had been trained. His knowledge of medicine, too, may have been quite regional. Maybe he felt that there was ONLY ONE WAY: HIS WAY! In any case, although the assistant registrar had inferred that things could be easily resolved, he was not the "BIG DOG" that the complaints chairman (now registrar) had enjoyed becoming. So I received a notice to practitioner that

- on or about March 21, 2001, you did examine the breasts of your patient, JM, when there was no medical reason for conducting that examination given the presenting complaint and history of your patient.

However, the college backed down on that one because they acknowledged that a complete medical would have been a very good reason to perform a breast exam; and

- on or about March 21, 2001, you did manipulate the nipples of the breasts of your patient, JM, in an effort to express secretions when there was no medical reason for doing that procedure given the presenting complaint and history of your patient.

They found that this allegation was proven because they were bamboozled. *You now know* something that the registrar, his surgical hitwoman, the hearing committee, and the Council of the College did not know: that this is taught in places that they know not of, as important aspects of a normal breast exam! Good for you!

2. <u>PV</u>:

This lady was a bit older than her friend JM. She had a child in school and a more-than-one-year-old child still breast-feeding. Please do not view that as a criticism from me of breast-feeding after age one. But you must understand that when it is still going on, the baby is almost never exclusively on breast-milk. Solids have virtually always been introduced, especially when there is a helpful older sibling. This makes quite a difference in determining what medications a mother can be put on. An infant completely dependent on breast milk will get more maternal medication than one who is on solids with "some" breast-feeding. I believe that the lawyer for the college or a medical advisor to him may have not understood this principle, with regard to low-dose lithium, and vilified me for it.

I attended this lady for counseling, prescribing, and medical care. I think she may not have seen me for much more than five to six months. She was referred by my psychologist friend. She had quite an entourage of support networks around her. She had my support. She was of my faith and had what most of you would call pastoral care through our church. She was seeing my psychologist friend. She had a social worker because she was on assistance. She had a life skills/career development helper from DECSA. I don't really know what training that person had. However, after I had attended PV for about six months, this DECSA helper called my office, asked to talk to me, and requested that I refer PV to a psychiatrist. Woe, now. Why was *she* asking me that? It would be a sixth "therapist" in the mix. And . . . why was the *career coach* doing the asking? I asked, "Are you a medically trained person?" She said no. I asked, "Then why are *you* making this request?" I was so surprised when she told me, "PV asked me to."

And I unfortunately spoke out loud my thoughts, "Why didn't she ask me herself? She must be . . . passive-aggressive!" I said it on the phone to this DECSA person. I assumed we were on the same team. *I assumed that we were both trying to help PV.* Maybe, she didn't even think she might be doing harm when she "gushed" to PV: "Your doctor called you passive-aggressive!" I guess for some, junior high school just never ends!

When PV saw me in a doorway a few days later, things had changed. She was no longer confident that she was in a trusting, working-together, professional relationship. Remember, this woman had been in four previous relationships, became pregnant, and had unsupported abortions and babies. The guys all panned. Just imagine her cumulative hurt. She'd become very sensitized to recognizing impending rejection. This time she felt it was coming from me.

So perhaps "enlightened" by JM's recounting of my past accusations, she phoned my office, spoke with my receptionist, and asked about *all of the times she had seen me* professionally and complained to the college about every one of them. Probably JM had told her the sordid tale of what the sexual assault center still thought of me. How sad. I wouldn't have rejected her as those other four men did, but I was not her boyfriend; I was a professional. We would have talked about addressing issues with appropriate individuals and not looking for a middleman – a Cirano de Bergerac. The claims she made were fairly vague, but the college managed to distill them down to sexual innuendo issues: *breast exam* in a lactating woman as a part of a medical, *and pelvic exam* as a part of an assessment for abdominal pain. She said that when she'd seen me for the abdominal pain, she had been worried about appendicitis. Maybe she had been. I don't remember. Someone referred during the hearing to the suggestion that I should have just focused on that possibility and ruled it in or out. But . . . my naïve friend . . . medicine is not practiced that way! Imagine the time that would be lost if we took one diagnosis and waited to disprove it before taking on another diagnosis in the same fashion. Medicine doesn't do that! Instead, we start with a history, add contributions from physical exam, and arrange investigations. If a person tells us that she has been lifting, cleaning house, and carrying heavy bottles some distance the day before her abdominal pain began, we already know that appendicitis is very, very unlikely. If we have the luxury of having the results of the most recent medical done just one month before, just under the page we are writing on, then we can SO EASILY refer to it. Information from it can reflect so much on what might be happening now. That really is a good way to help the diagnostic process.

Reader, you already know about the college accusations of inappropriate breast expression (when I was looking for adenitis) and repeating a vaginal exam after laxatives in order to be sure that one is examining each ovary instead of a lump of stool. After she stopped seeing me, for a time, PV moved on to another Edmonton doctor who did send her to a psychiatrist in the Edmonton area. She was again *content, BRIEFLY,* with her emotional connections (though her emotional connections were almost all professional because she couldn't manage other types). She then moved back to New Brunswick. Perhaps she is changing doctors there, even now as you read. She was not well taught by whomever she saw subsequently and believed that I should have, in retrospect, been doing sequential blood work on her when I was prescribing "such high doses of lithium" to her (page 108, lines 15 and on to page 109). Of course, 300 to 600 mg per night, as an augmenting agent and mood stabilizer, are *not high doses* and almost never require lab work. And by the way, I have treated with 2100–2700 mg of lithium, and certainly in these *higher* doses, regular blood work is necessary! With whom did you speak, PV? I sincerely suggest that you try to stick with just one main prescriber/provider. That person needs your help in order to figure out the right treatment for you. Sometimes you might be upset with your doctor. None of us are magical. None of us can treat you without involving you. And yes, that includes figuring out that you have passive-aggressive traits. That is not a condemnation but a diagnosis, girl. Work it through.

3. WG:

The way the college dealt with this lady's complaint is what disappointed me most about them. I was perplexed. I didn't know if they actually believed any part of what she said, or if they just used her complaint as a vehicle for some personal vendetta. I lost faith in my profession through their dealings about her. I had felt that the college was an ethical guide to the profession. It just wasn't . . . for me! It really may have done some good work, if heavy-handed, with others. But on with WG!

The tale doesn't begin with the incident of 30 December 2001, but over a long string of contacts that I have found, I had had with her for several years before. All of these had been at the XXXX General Hospital. Most of the contacts had been for migraine headache. She had been there so often that it would not take much to fabricate a "recollection" of one of those migraine-type hospital visits. When she had come 31 October 1998, in my assessment of possible contributing factors to her migraine, I found cervical vertebral somatic dysfunction. I explained my findings to her and also explained that I could possibly overcome her migraine headache with manual therapy to her neck. Because she was feeling terrible, she agreed to let me try. I did the neck manipulation and could feel the resolution of the somatic dysfunction in her neck. She told me that her migraine was gone! Without meds! We had proven two things:

1. the final common pathway or unification theory of migraine and that subtracting one contributor to the complex can make a distinct difference.
2. And that I did manual therapy.

However, as is true for many interventions, the muscles that had shortened wanted to pull things back out of position. And a while later, her neck again was very stiff. She called my office on the 19 November 1998 and demanded that I *undo* what I had done. Now this was nineteen days after treatment. On the phone, she agreed that my treatment had removed her migraine. It was the "new" neck stiffness that she was upset about. I agreed to assess her either at my office as early as the next day or in emerg when next I was there. I didn't see her again for this. I suppose that she saw physiotherapy and did heating packs with or without muscle relaxants for a time. The truth is that I had forgotten about her by December 2001. But *she could hardly have forgotten* about me. I did see her in January 1999 for left maxillary sinusitis, which can also cause headache but needs an antibiotic, not manual therapy or potent pain medications.

Then I saw her again at the XXXX General Hospital in the very wee hours of 30 December 2001. This time it wasn't for migraine. She complained of lower back discomfort to (1) the lady at the registration desk. She complained of lower back pain going down one leg to (2) the nurse who took her into the examination room. She couldn't/wouldn't sit down. She complained to (3) me of pain in her right low back, jabbing right down to her right toes. She told me (as a part of her history) that these jolts happened about each half to one hour and had been present for the preceding four days. She explained that seven weeks ago, she'd had a fall with head injury, loss of consciousness, and "broken tailbone." I specifically wrote her next phrase to me, "I'm not sure why I'm here 'cause you can't fix a tailbone." A broken tailbone is, of course, a lay term with NO specific medical meaning. She told me that she'd also had ten to twelve shots of Demerol in the preceding seven weeks for headaches since the fall. She said she's tried (1) Demerol tablets, that (2) Percocet worked but made her need to sleep more, and that she had (3) Fiorinal capsules. All in all, a lovely mix of very potent pain meds. She said she'd been menopausal for the last three months. She was forty-six years old, was married, and had children.

I left the room after taking her history and brought her back a gown and a half sheet with which to cover herself. I asked that she remove her clothing and her bra but suggested that she could keep her panties on. I found the nurse who was working emerg with me, and we waited in the hallway for a time to allow her to finish changing. Then *we went in together* for the examination. I did an assessment on her. I ruled out disc protrusion sciatica by exam. She is always a chatterer, and this time was not different. I deduced that she had a sciatica-like syndrome. In the midst of her chatting away, she may not have heard all that I explained to her, and the nurse who was chaperoning for me could also reasonably have missed things. Really, only a court reporter would have the discipline to get it all down and might well have had to use tapes for review.

The course of my examination led me to consider a mass (abscess or tumor) pushing on the nerves OR a muscle through which the sciatic nerve passed being shortened or tightened. And I still had no idea *what she meant* by a "broken tailbone." Was some posttraumatic event making the piriformis muscle compress the sciatic nerve? I had previously brought her that hospital gown and half sheet with which to drape herself. Before going on to determine what therapy might be appropriate, I informed her that I needed to do a pelvic exam to check the pelvic floor. The anterior superior iliac spine was high on the left, but the right sciatic notch and right SI joint were tender. Her jolting electrical pain was going down the right leg. On which side should I focus which therapy?

I asked that she remove her panties so that we could do a pelvic exam to determine the main side of injury, as both were suspect. When I provide information to a patient, he/she understands about 7 percent of what I say. It's not that I speak badly (I hope), but this is true of all communication: 7 percent words, perhaps 37 percent intonation, and 56 percent body language. Those that stipulate the need for elaborate verbal communication just don't know much about how it is received. Really, a visualization in the form of a video has proven to be the most effective to give information that can allow consent to a procedure or intervention. We don't ever have those just sitting in the emergency room, waiting to be used.

While she slipped off her underwear and got into the lithotomy position, the nurse held up the half sheet to provide her some privacy. She could not see me but may have assumed that I was there while she took off her underthings. The nurse, I suspect, was looking at her in order to prevent private things from being in open display. (HH, you did that very well every time I worked with you.) I stepped back out of the curtained cubicle and fetched a glove and lubricant: it would have taken me literally seconds to return. Neither of them might have seen me go and come. They were each occupied. When she was ready, I sat on the bed just beyond her buttocks. I then asked that she assume the traditional "frog leg" position, medically called lithotomy.

I checked the pelvic floor, found no dominant mass (tumor or abscess), found no abnormal anteversion in the coccygeal chain of bones (and I suspect I am the only physician in Alberta who knows that of her – and, in truth, when I touched the perhaps still bruised coccyx, it may have *hurt*), but then I found the right but not left pubococcygeus muscle to be like the thickest string on a bass fiddle. There was my answer. She says that she cried out in pain not just once but a second time (with the plucking of the pubococcygeus). I have no recollection of that specifically, but I have felt that very tight pubococcygeus band of muscle and seen <u>pain</u> associated with it several other times.

She also says that when she got home, she noted vaginal blood. I can say without equivocation that virtually every physician on earth looks at his glove or gloves after an exam. I know I do. For two reasons: to make sure that the glove is still sound (doesn't have a hole in it) and to examine the glove for the color of rectal or vaginal secretions. I would have noted it on the chart if there were blood, and there was NONE. I would have run to the sink to wash if there was a hole. I would also have used a notation on the chart right then that I had been exposed to the bodily fluids of a person with unknown infectious disease status. This is to enable follow-up for possible exposure to hepatitis viruses and HIV.

After having made a diagnosis of *right* piriformis syndrome (although I did write *left* piriformis syndrome, on the chart – I'm admitting a mistake there], I asked the patient to assist me in seeing whether her problem could be overcome with manual therapy. I would have explained that I had received training in this regard and believed I might be able to help her. But of course, I would not know that she *already knew that* from my previous treatment to her neck. Given that the previous treatment did not produce satisfying results, why would she not jump up and say, "No way! Not again!" However, she cooperated with me while I did three manipulations. That means that she listened to me and moved into the positions that I requested. The first was to attempt to reduce the high left ASIS (anterior superior iliac spine) with a long leg "tug." We then checked to see if the ASISs were now at equal heights. They were, so we had appropriately dealt with the left innominate upslip (hemipelvis being driven up in an impact). Do I actually recall this being the case? No, but I would *not have gone on if the ASIS was still high*. Upon recheck, the tenderness to the right sciatic notch was still there, though. So we rechecked the tissue tone beside the lower lumbar vertebrae and found the right side to be denser.

This is consistent with a right-sided lumbar somatic dysfunction. Therefore, we attempted a long-lever maneuver of the lumbar spine with her lying on her left side. I would have used the nurse to help me with this maneuver, to help keep the patient's extended straight left leg from slipping off the table. Then we rechecked again. She complained to the committee that she kept asking, "Is all of this necessary?" And yes, rechecks are necessary in doing a sequence of manual therapies. Unfortunately, the right sciatic notch was still tender. So we tried simply stretching her right piriformis muscle using a muscle-energy technique. I would like to be able to say that made her completely better. But there was still some tenderness to the right sciatic notch, so she was *only partially better* – by my reassessments. At that point, I would have stopped attempts at manual intervention. (Most of us stop at about three.) And I prescribed drugs. She told me that nonsteroidal anti-inflammatories (NSAIDs) caused her blood in the stool, so I wrote Vioxx, which is a COX II inhibitor and Flexeril (an effective muscle relaxant) for her for fifteen days. We gave her the first dose while she was there in the hospital because we wanted to get her started, and *she certainly had no contraindication, such as nausea or vomiting*. Before leaving, she asked what she might do about the increased tendency for migraines to occur. At that point, as a favor to her, I did an abbreviated head and neck exam for her – she was back in her street clothing, by this time. I noted that her right temperomandibular joint clicked but was not tender, that the muscles of mastication were not tender, that the temporal arteries were not tender and pulsed normally, that she had a normal three fingertip opening of the jaw, and that there was a distinct right occipital neuritic tenderness. This means that when I palpated it in its notch on the right but not the left side, she got head pain from where I was touching, jabbing forward into her right face, especially around the eye. I informed her of my findings. I told her that I or someone else with the skills could inject the area around that right occipital nerve with a local anaesthetic and steroid and probably cause the headaches to vanish for from six weeks to perhaps forever.

She, like many, probably didn't much like the idea of getting a needle in the back of the head/neck, but she seemed to appreciate my information. We said good night. The nurse at the desk noticed that she was happier and walking more easily as she left. I had had the other nurse, HH, in with me the whole time of the assessment and interventions. We parted on good terms.

Now I am going to write out for you her letter of complaint written *three days after* our encounter. She had already conferred with her lawyer, which I initially thought was very quick; but since finding out that she sues multiple people and organizations, I don't now consider it at all surprising. She could probably get quickly connected to that lawyer – speed dial! Here is her written complaint in all its splendor:

"Dear Sharon (Barron)

Further to our conversation of today, please accept the following as my account of the incident of December 30, 2001.

At approximately 12:00-1:00 am on December 30th I attended the emergency department of the XXXX General Hospital. I was following instructions from my family physician regarding an injury that occurred on October 24, 2001. I had fallen, bounced my head off a concrete sidewalk and landed on the edge of a curb, leaving myself with a fractured tailbone and rendering myself unconscious. [She, of course, sued the proprietor of the place with the icy surface.]

"I was taken to hospital in Edmonton where I was treated and released under the observation of my family physician. Since I have been suffering with migraine headaches due to the onset of menopause and a hormonal change, this injury was affecting those headaches due to the muscle swelling and pressure on the nerves in my neck and lower back. I have been examined and treated and also attend therapy for this injury. The Fiorinol, which was prescribed for me, does not always work, due to the severity of the migraines. My physician was on holidays and before he left, his instructions were, 'If the pain becomes too severe, *go to the hospital and get a shot*,' (which I have done previously), *for the pain* of migraines."

[OK, now this is me adding a question: From these first sixteen lines of her complaint letter, what is it that this patient believes she has a right to when now going to emerg? This isn't sneaky, I have the phrase underlined. It's a "shot for pain," right? She thinks it is her right to have a "shot for pain." That's what we get from her letter so far. There are a total of 146 lines in the letter. We have looked at sixteen of them. Let's go on.]

"I explain this to you first Sharon, because I also explained this all to Dr Litchfield before he began his examination. When I first arrived, I went to admissions and explained that I had a migraine, likely aggravated by an injury to my tailbone. The attending nurse wrote, 'lower back injury' (???) on my chart and gave it to Dr Litchfield. I explained the situation to him as soon as he came in to see me to make it clear as to the purpose of my visit." [My insert: And the purpose of her visit was? "To get my shot for pain." So the gist of the first twenty-two lines of this letter is to emphasize that she was here to get her shot for pain.]

"He was sitting at the bedside taking notes as I explained this to him, so I assume he heard me. With no word, he left the cubicle we were in, returned within a moment or so with a gown [notice that she doesn't say "a gown and a sheet"] that had been previously worn (it was wrinkled and had a long black hair caught in the tie), instructing me to 'take off my things.' I asked him, 'Why do I have to take my clothes off *for a migraine?*' He simply left the area. I removed my clothes (except I left my underpants and socks on) as instructed." [My comment: Well, now it's getting a bit more intriguing, isn't it? The thrust of this paragraph is that I didn't communicate much, and despite what little I had said, she knew enough to remove *clothing that would be in the way of a back exam.* If she were, as she says, there for a migraine, then why did she remove her blouse and bra?

She clearly still maintained some choices because she kept her underpants and socks on. Why did she choose to remove her slacks, her shirt, and her bra that would enable her back to be seen . . . but for a migraine? Does this seem likely?]

"An attendant (nurse, short reddish hair, glasses) came in, took my blood pressure, asked me if I normally had high blood pressure. I said, 'No, only when I have this terrible pain for so long.' She told me my blood pressure was 'quite high,' and noted it on my chart I believe. 'It won't be long,' she said. 'You look like you are in pain. The doctor will be in very soon.' I thanked her and she left." [My note: Now it becomes more plain. The person at the desk had actually brought her to the room and had taken her pulse, respiratory rate, temperature, and oxygen saturations – but not the blood pressure! That's why I had to do it and entered it clearly on the chart in *my writing*. So this *paragraph* is completely bogus, made-up (perhaps from a recall of past emergency room visits, and she has had a lot of them). This little add-on is, perhaps, to boost the prominence of her "migraine severity." But she had not come with a migraine.]

"Dr Litchfield returned just after that and walked into my cubicle. He walked right to me (after placing my chart on the counter). I was sitting against the bed, but had my feet on the black stool beside the bed. Dr Litchfield asked me to sit up on the bed. I did. He went around behind me, reached up under the gown I was wearing and ran his hand over my right breast, lightly squeezing it and then to the middle of my chest where he pushed as he held my back in the same place (???). He brushed past my breast again as he removed his hand. *A nurse walked into the cubicle at this point.*" [Now what is wrong with this paragraph? Well, she says she was *sitting against* the bed and then with my prompt she *sat* up on the bed – but the staff had noted her to be *unwilling to sit* at the registration desk and very reluctant to sit in the cubicle because of her *sore "tailbone."* But let's suppose we could believe the less believable, and here she is sitting on the hospital bed. Now let me ask you, where are the flaps of her hospital gown? If you're a woman, you'll know the answer – *she is sitting on them*! Like every woman in every hospital in the entire world! Then, certainly, the next part becomes more technically difficult: how do you reach up under the gown that a chubby woman is sitting on – *without knocking her off the flaps*, first? Further, the nurse in question agrees that we waited outside the curtained cubicle until we were confident that she had changed, and then *ENTERED TOGETHER*! It's starting to sound like a country/Western song: "So if she says that this has happened trust me girl when I say she's lyin' agin."]

"He then instructed me to stand. I did. He asked me to bend over in front of him while he sat on a stool. I felt very uncomfortable bending over a foot from him in my underpants, but he insisted I try." [Sorry, I was trying to wait 'til the end of the paragraph, but I just couldn't. So here is a woman who has just described having her breast fondled and has said nothing but goes on to feel "very uncomfortable bending over"! Really? And just a foot from me? Did you knock me in the face with your underpants-covered bum? Reader, do you find this tale is sounding a bit fishy?] "My head was pounding; I felt nauseous and had been vomiting already. I refused to bend over any further." [This suggests that she still did possess some assertiveness, so why was it absent when she was being groped?] "He said something I did not understand and then asked me to lay on the bed. At this point I don't remember everywhere he touched in detail. I know he poked and prodded at my hips and my sides. He pressed his thumbs into the front of my pubic area" [Actually, right on the pubic tubercles where some inner thigh muscles attach.] "that hurt!" [On one side or both?] He pressed on my stomach and seemed to be measuring my legs." [She is almost accurate here – we're looking at the ASISs (anterior superior iliac spines) which border each side of the low abdomen.] "He was straightening them out. He then, as I was lying on back, pulled my gown up and reached between my breasts again and pushed on my chest and ran his fingers (2 or 3) in short rapid motions, down the front of my chest and abdomen, right down to my pubic area (???)."

[She's not even close to accurate here, and *this did not happen*. It sounds more like a piano concerto like my mother used to do.] "I was in pain and did not think any of this was necessary. When he pushed his thumbs into the creases at the top of my legs, I said, 'Did you have any friends when you were a kid?'" [Ah, the humor! And I do remember that because it really was funny – it stands out!] I was attempting to, in good humor, let him know I was not impressed with this examination [So to her, cute humorous phrases are meant to convey displeasure and anger at having been assaulted?], and his prodding. He said nothing. The nurse acknowledged me. She was continually covering me up.

Dr Litchfield then asked me to lie on my stomach. I did so. He then ran his thumbs up my spine, down my bum area and asked me to lie on my back again. At this point, I said, 'Is this necessary?' (???) I looked at the nurse (dark hair, glasses) and she shrugged her shoulders. He pulled my underpants down to the top of my legs at the back [it is imperative (to her civil suit) that she verbalize something apparently assaultive or violent] and repeated his "examination" of my behind. I reached down and pull up my pants.

He then asked me to roll over onto my back and lie flat, which is very uncomfortable for me without my knees up due to the tailbone injury." [Aha! Now we get her take on the pain of the tailbone! So it wasn't sore when she was sitting with her feet up on the black stool, or when I asked her to sit up in bed – as it would be to every other living being with an injured "tailbone" – while I fondled the breast.

She wants us to accept that it really only now hurt, with her lying down. Wow! Has she not at least looked up the pain-aggravating factors for tailbone injury when she made up this complaint?] "Then with no warning, Dr Litchfield pulled my underpants down [again, the aura of violence] and began pushing on areas of my pelvis again. I reached down to pull them back up because I felt uncomfortable [At this point? Really?] and Dr Litchfield said, 'You will have to take these off.' I asked, 'Why?' and he just motioned to the nurse as though she was to carry out his instructions." [What "motion" is that?] "I pulled my underpants off while objecting and still lying on my back, trying to stay covered (this nice nurse was holding the sheet up like you would a bath towel to change behind). I objected to his *standing at the foot of the bed*, opening my legs and looking between them. I said, 'My *head* is throbbing, is this necessary?' [You see she is still maintaining that she was there for a migraine. The nurse at the desk said back pain, the nurse that took her into the examination room said back pain going down the right leg, and I said that she came for back pain radiating down the right leg. But the three of us are wrong? And she is right? We know she had been to emerg thirty to forty times for migraine, perhaps twenty times that year. She wants us to believe that she was such a novice at being examined for migraine, that she would actually ask if a pelvic exam were necessary for her migraine, *this time*?] "As I finished that, *without any warning* whatsoever, Dr Litchfield shoved his fingers of one hand up into my vagina, and pushed on my pubic bone with his other hand." [Again, she conveys violence.]

[When I do a pelvic exam on a patient in a hospital bed, I always sit on the right side of the bed just beyond the patient's buttocks. I then allow the patient to gently assume the lithotomy position. We know this patient is lying, and we know that she is lying to promote her civil litigation against me and against the Regional Health Authority (because they have more money than I do), so potential big settlement money is possible. She is hoping to win the big lawsuit lottery. With the slipping on ice thing, she has made money. The broken toilet seat scam she has perfected. She is a con woman. So we're going to interrupt her letter with an insert from her evidence at the disciplinary hearing. I promise we'll get right back to her strangely crafted letter after this. Here's what she said verbally about this pelvic exam, "under oath."]

Page 202: "At this point, Dr Litchfield took a hold of both my knees with his hands, and he opened my legs, and that's the point where this examination was not okay with me anymore [so was the initial groping which you claim happened at the beginning, okay with you?], because in my own description, I have had three children, and I have never had somebody else take my knees and open my legs like that before, and I felt uncomfortable with him *standing at the foot of my bed doing that . . .*" [Oops! Lies don't hang together very well! Here is what she proposes I was doing – standing at the foot of her bed pressing her knees apart, . . . from there, . . . from the foot of the bed! At that point, I was not doing yoga, but even now that I do yoga, I cannot do that. But wait, it gets better. Try to comprehend this that follows.] Page 203: "The next thing I remember is when I had my knees up, and I said: Is this necessary, he had opened my legs, I thought he was going to manipulate again with his thumbs or do whatever he was doing, and the next thing I know, he shoved his fingers inside of me, and he scratched me [with his latex glove; WG, are you mixing this up with your recall of "<u>Hook</u>," that story about Peter Pan?], and I remember yelping because it hurt, and I had a headache, and I felt that in my head at the same time, and I said: Ow, that hurt, and he said: Sorry, and he did it again; and at that point, I pulled my legs together, and I remember I had tears rolling down my face [but no one else remembers that], because I was in pain. I was feeling like this wasn't necessary. Why did this have to happen? I trusted this doctor," [Would this trust have been given a real boost when I messed up your neck for nineteen days, three years before?] "and yet, I was feeling very violated, and, like, this didn't have to happen, and what did it have to do with my head?" [WG, *if only you knew how much this façade has to do with your head!*]

"So I tried to get up off the bed, and I swung my legs around to try and get up off the bed to the left, and when I did, Dr Litchfield had come around to the side of the bed, and he sat here right on my right-hand side on the bed . . ." [Oh my goodness! This implies_*that I did the PELVIC EXAM from the foot of the bed* too! Sorry, lady, my arms aren't nearly that long, and I have a back that would never let me bend that far forward from the foot of the bed in question. Are you thinking of Elastigirl in the *Incredibles*? Really, when you lie to pursue a con game, you really need to do more homework. Did you ever see *The Sting*? Do some choreography, girl! Nevertheless, picking up on the next theme of her letter of complaint (and no longer her evidence under oath at the hearing)]: "I attempted to get up when Dr Litchfield came around to the side of the bed and" [Finally, I was becoming sooooo exhausted with all that stretching] "sat down on the bed beside me. He instructed me to lie on my side, and then proceeded to lift my legs (together) and pull them around the front of him, on his lap with my bare buttocks up against his side and my gown falling off me. He pushed my one leg over the other until I felt I would fall of the bed. I said then, 'Are you a Chiropractor or something? Enough!' He said, 'I make no claim to chiropractic medicine, but I do practice osteopathic medicine and they are sometimes related.' I asked what this had to do with my headache and he simply said, 'You can get dressed,' and walked out. The nurse helped me onto my feet and she left also.

"I dressed and remained in the cubicle, feeling more intense pain than when I had arrived. The nurse returned to check on me. I asked if the doctor was going to treat me? [She implies that manual therapy is not treatment.] She opened the curtain saying, 'I don't know yet, I'll see.'

I followed her out the door to the main desk where Dr Litchfield was standing. I had been in the examination room directly across from the desk. It was only a few steps. He saw me and said, 'I'm going to give you an anti-inflammatory and a muscle relaxant and I want you to keep working, but only eight to ten hours a day, no more.' (???)

"I told him I could not take *most* anti-inflammatory medications, as I have an ulcer due to the chemicals in the last dose I was prescribed and told him they make my stomach bleed, and that they do not help relieve the migraine. He totally disregarded my statement and said, 'Have you had Vioxx before?' [Not a traditional anti-inflammatory.] I said, 'Yes.' He then instructed the nurse (I believe) to get me two (2) Vioxx and two (2) Flexeril tablets. She went for them and returned with an envelope and instructions. I was still standing there, *complaining of the blinding light*' [WG, why had you not brought your dark glasses to the hospital for your claimed photophobia, this time?] "when she returned. As I was apparently being *dismissed* by Dr Litchfield, paying no regard to the headache I was suffering, I said, 'Can't you give me anything for this migraine?' He said, 'I think we need to deal with the muscle injury and spasm first.' (???) He then said, 'Here is a prescription for 25 [well, 15] days (or so),' and walked away.

"I was humiliated and left in more severe pain than when I arrived. I walked to the foyer, I crouched down to my knees inside the main entrance and cried. I felt violated. I was hurt. I had a blinding migraine. My blood pressure was throbbing in *my throat* [Oh really. *Your throat? Not in one temple*, like migraine pulses or throbs in the other 150 million migraine sufferers in the world?] and I was *nearly* photophobic [but what about the blinding light thing?] from the pain and light. I was nauseous to the point of gagging." [So do you think you could easily swallow oral medications and keep them down? See, below.]

"I stood up to leave, went outside and toward my van. As I was walking, Dr Litchfield walked up beside me (about ten feet away) walking toward another vehicle. I looked at him and said, 'Why did you have to do that to me?' He simply kept walking, as he said, 'Have a nice evening.' (???) [So here she expects to be believed that this terrible doctor had abused her horribly in that bad hospital and she wanted to get away from him and that place so badly that she struck up a conversation with him in the otherwise *empty parking lot in the sheer darkness* of approximately 01:30 hours in the morning. That seems likely doesn't it? Chefs do that, right?]

"I arrived at my van where I called my daughter who arrived with my son to take me home approximately 15 minutes later. As I sat there in pain waiting, it seemed much longer. When I arrived home and changed for bed, I noticed I had fresh blood spots on the lining of my underpants and in hindsight wondered if Dr Litchfield had been wearing a glove when he scratched me. I don't remember him putting gloves on or leaving the area to do so." [Now this "*he wasn't wearing gloves*" is a claim from the 1989 newspapers when accusations against me were first made public. The inference is that a physician trained in infection and disease would want to expose himself regularly to avoidable human body fluids. WG, are you doing a "me too, me too"?]

"I spent the night and early morning vomiting, retching, and in horrible pain until my mother arrived with 50 mg Demerol and Gravol [so these were taken by mouth]. It took a total of six Demerol, taken two at a time, to relieve the pain enough *for me to function*." [And if you had been so, so nauseated, why did you *not throw these up?*] "I spent the better part of the next 12 hours sleeping off the Demerol and Gravol." [But you just said you *could function*, and now you're saying that you *couldn't* because of the somnolence. Which is it?] "I had five New Year's Eve parties to decorate for our clients . . . I am a decorator and I should have been in my shoppe. I had to have staff do what I should have been there to do. I feel *all this could have been avoided* had Dr Litchfield simply acted in accordance with the immediate problem, e.g. the migraine and the vomiting." [So she is right back at the "I deserved a shot" theme.] "I *worked* all New Year's Eve day, 'hungover' from the drugs [except for the part, that you spent sleeping off the drugs, right?] and was too sick to join my family (children) on New Year's Eve.

"I called the hospital and spoke to the nurse the night after this incident. She remembered me and the 'incident' that happened. She encouraged me to write a letter of complaint to Pat Brakey (who I believe is the hospital administrator) and gave me the address of the College of Physicians and Surgeons. She suggested I send 'them' a copy. She 'didn't want to say too much more' (I understand).

"I have reported this incident to my family physician, XXXX. He also agreed that in a situation such as the one I reported, a doctor would treat the immediate problem and then with a follow up exam perhaps later if he felt it was necessary. He agreed I should document this account and report it.

"This is my [ever so creative and "bid for the gold"] account of the events of this incident. I feel I was violated, and not informed of the doctor's intentions, or given warning of his intention to enter my body, refusal of immediate and necessary treatment and blatant disregard of my requests and objections to this examination procedure. I now fear the possibility of having been infected internally as well." [This last – *"oh my, I might be infected"* is another direct 1989 media quote from the issues that brought the 1992 and 1996 trials. No need to strain for personal originality here, WG!]

So this lady who props up her decorating business with financial settlements from ongoing litigations is saying she went in with her usual migraine, and that awful doctor-man did a bunch of investigations and treatments on me as if I had come in with right-sided back pain radiating down the right leg. *The two nurses and the doctor were all wrong* in thinking that I came in because of back and leg pain. I am right, and those three – although they are in agreement – are wrong! And the fine committee tried to buy into this garbage complaint.

Now listen, WG. You've still got a civil suit against me. Do you think that a real live judge is not going to recognize the so-familiar-to-him disharmony of your perjury? He will have you serving prison time for it. But if you are still *addicted to danger* in playing out a con/fraud, then bring it on, girl!

Are you really going to tell us this tripe and yet claim to be an addictions counselor? You and I know that most addictions counselors get into the field because they have had an addiction, right? So are you *substituting addictions*: an addiction for narcotics or alcohol for an addiction to danger through fraud? Really, where are you at in your recovery? Where do steps 8 and 9 fit into your twelve-step program – willingness to make amends and then making them. If this is never a part of your recovery, how will you possibly help others overcome their addictions?

4. PF:

This lady is the wife of the pastor in one of the churches in XXXX. Her husband is the pastor to WG. WG works within his church organization as a drug and alcohol counselor for teens possibly. Wow! This is a tight-knit group. She had had an assessment by me on the first of September 2001. She wrote the date of her complaint letter as February 23, 2002. However, it was stamped as received by the college on January 28, 2002, and I received a copy of it with a cover letter from the college complaints investigator dated February 13, 2002. She is the one for whom the nurse who acted as chaperone for me could not be found – at least by the Counsel for the College, upon whose honor my lawyer seems to have relied. Then, she was just so easily found because she still worked regularly at the XXXX hospital. You'll remember that I've said that when the chairman of the hearing committee confronted the college counsel, *as a representative of the college*, about why she could not be found, he said his ever-so-revealing (page 289 of second transcript) *"I have no explanation."* Pardon me, counsel, what was that explanation? Did you say that as a lawyer admitted to the Bar of the Province of Alberta, upon whose word my lawyer relied, your answer is, *"I have no explanation"*! When you are questioned by the bar association, will that still be your answer? And do you expect that that will be believed?

Still, let me present the complaint letter of PF because there are more than two witnesses whose statements were not truthful in my disciplinary hearing. Here goes,

> Alberta College of Physicians and Surgeons
> Attention: Sharron Barron February 23, 2002
>
> On September 1, 2001, I was admitted to the Emergency Department of the XXXX General Hospital for treatment of a migraine headache. A nurse took me to an emergency room and recorded medical information. Dr Bryant Litchfield was the doctor on call. He asked me why I was there. I told him I had a migraine headache. He checked my neck and jaw. Then he asked me to stand up because he had to check my back. He lifted up my sweatshirt and asked permission to undo my bra. I responded, "I guess so." He then asked me to bend forward, slipped his hands underneath my bra. He touched my breasts and moved his bare arms around my chest. He said he had to get closer, so he squeezed between the bed and myself pulling me backwards until I could feel his body on my bum and legs. He backed away asking me which closure I used on my bra, offering to do it up. I said it was okay I would do it up myself. He then proceeded to

prescribe medication. I would greatly appreciate it if you would handle this matter for me.

Sincerely,
PF

There it is. Seventeen lines in this text; I think I might have said fourteen earlier. Now, reader, as you go through this, can you get the exact sequence of things? Do you know precisely what is being complained of? Well, neither did I. Is she saying that I had her stand up, lifted up her shirt, with permission undid her bra, asked her to bend over, then slipped my hands onto her breasts, and pulled her into me so that the front of me was rubbing into her bum and legs, *all at once*? And this would be *in front of the nurse* who was there chaperoning? That must have been some very engrossing "charting" to keep her from noticing this sordid scene! And then I just asked if I should close her bra, wrote a prescription, and we parted? Is that what she was describing? Is that even remotely possible? *Does this lady or her husband have a collection of pornography because this story line is very cheap and risqué* and has a D budget (or worse) screenplay. Don't you have some questions that you would like this complainant to elaborate on? Would you not want to be sure of every detail here? The college investigator received the letter but didn't "apparently" EVER interview her. She instead asked for my written reply to the accusation letter specifically with regard to allegations of

- inappropriate physical boundaries and
- unhooking the patient's bra.

No mention of putting each hand on a breast and pulling her into my body with her bent over at the time? PF later says that the breast contact lasted one to two minutes, not longer than two minutes! Oh my gosh! But the "investigator" didn't read it that way, so asked me to comment on the *unclasping of the bra* (which you will learn is a standard taught in the only physicians boundaries course in our country) and *"getting too close"* to the patient. I certainly hoped to get further information about this possibly clumsy, possibly sexual assaultive narrative. We really need the exact details, don't we?

Well, I wrote her back on the twenty-eight of February 2002:

Dear Ms D.

I am in receipt of the letter of complaint of PF dated February 23, 2002 but received by the College 28 Jan 2002. This lady is, I trust we can agree, a friend or church acquaintance of WG. She has chosen nine days after my hospital privileges were suspended in January 2002, to lodge her complaint about an encounter on September 1, 2001 at the XXXX General Hospital – five months before.

We will not need to refer to the timing of this complaint as coincidental. Nevertheless, I find the tone of her letter to be very forth right [if vague] and do not [yet] sense any embellishment on her behalf. I do not disagree with any part of what she reports and will in my description of events touch on all that she writes, and more.

Ms F registered at the desk at 13:59 hrs on Saturday the first of September, 2001. I see that I recorded her 'away time' as 16:38 hrs, so it was probably a while between registration and actually being seen: it must have been busy. I do not specifically recall this encounter with Ms F but I know that she is the wife of one of the local pastors, and it is possible that I have attended her in *emergency* previously.

Mostly I am using my notes and my awareness of my routine to recreate this scenario.

1. She told the desk she was there to be seen for migraine.
2. Her physician routinely was Dr XXXX.

3. A staff nurse had written her as allergic to Penicillin and aspirin, had listed six medications that she took but not their dosages, and had provided a sketchy overview of her reason for being there. In fact, I recognize the signature as Gaina Brooker's (the nurse) [who couldn't be found].

4. I don't know which cubicle she was in (the two in the large room are more spacious than the five in the other room) and this may have been a factor. [The number of stretchers in each room has changed many times over the years. I worked *emergency* here, in 1988–92, and then 1996-2002. They had adequate local staff in the interim. The rooms were very adaptable, in part because this emergency department didn't ever use the hallways. It was one of the things I liked about the place. However, when the area was full I believe that there could be a total of seven beds or stretchers in the combined two rooms. Those days we worked in tight quarters. It is possible that such was the situation when PF came that day.]

5. She says that a nurse came in with me but that *may* not be correct especially on a busy day. I *might* only have gone for the nurse when I'd finished taking my own history. [I loved working with the fine nurses in XXXX. They were professional yet friendly and welcoming. As of 1989, when I was portrayed by the media as one of America's Most Wanted, we all knew the score – huge allegations had been made about me. I spoke with the chief of staff at that rural hospital. I didn't want to bring a bad reputation to that fine place. I was told that my medical work was fine and that the nurses liked working with me. They completely supported my insistence on having a chaperone for every female patient who needed the curtains closed for her visit. That's how we worked. Some of them seemed quite interested in the manual therapy techniques that I was acquiring. They

didn't snooze in a chair. They didn't bring charting into the exam room to keep themselves busy. They watched. They were alert. They often asked questions after a patient encounter. To say that any one of them was casual or inattentive is to cast aspersions that are wrongful and malicious about those fine nurses.]

6. She elaborated for me the dosages of the medications:
    - Zoloft 100 mg BID
    - Deseryl 75 mg @ HS
    - Maxeran ½ hr before each meal
    - Didrocal [this is taken once daily]
    - Epival 150 mg BID, and
    - Estraderm (an estrogen patch)

7. She said she'd been struggling with depression, that she was not employed, that she lived with her husband and that "these headaches (bad) been keeping me from normal life".

8. She told me that "lately they've (doctors) been giving me Demerol, Gravol & DHE" but she did not provide dosages the way a drug-seeker might. There is a "frequent visitor" book at the desk but I don't know if she is in it.

9. She said that she'd been on the *Estrogen patch* since November for hot flashes – of course, Estrogens can be associated with increased headache, but more especially combined *estrogens by mouth*.

10. She informed me that she had had a right stiff shoulder since the previous September – about one year before.

11. She knew something of migraines and told me (probably sheepishly) that she had had cheese the day before. [Old cheese, red wine, some beers, chocolate, MSG, bisulphites, and shellfish all seem to be migraine triggers for some.]

12. She explained that she had awakened that morning with vomiting, diarrhea, blurred vision (and headache, though I didn't need to write that) at 05:00 hrs.

13. It was clear this was not a singular, new, sudden onset headache, nor one associated with a diminished level of consciousness: there was a familiar pattern. [A headache that is very different from a patient's usual headache pattern can spell real danger, and needs investigation usually with diagnostic imaging (like a CT Scan).]

14. At this point, I would be ready to examine and would seek a nurse if one was not there. I don't dispute Gaiana may have already been there – she herself has migraine disorder herself, and I have treated her several times: she may have been interested.

15. I found her blood pressure to be 100/78 on the right with her sitting. [This is very reassuring in an acute headache situation.] I recorded the heart rate at 86/min.

16. I did a head and neck exam. If she was really photophobic, I wouldn't press for fundoscopy [eye exam with a bright light] in this particular instance. I put my hands through her collar (as I always do) and palpated her neck muscles and trapezii – these I found very, very tight.

17. I palpated the temporalis and masseter muscles and found these not tender or tight. The TMJs (tempero-mandibular joints) were also not tender to palpation during opening and closing of the mouth. At this point I would check the oral opening and confirm 3 finger tips could pass between her teeth. Though I did not record this I do not doubt that I did it and that the response was normal.

18. I checked her range of neck motion and found it to be restricted in every direction – but not painful. This, I call a capsular pattern (symmetrical limitations not worse on one side). [The fact that there is no pain on neck movement is also very important. A viral meningitis might well present as a headache, but there is often pain to the movement of the neck especially flexion and extension.]

19. In this particular lady, I would be in error not to check the upper back and peripectoral muscle tone – given her complaint of a frozen shoulder, the chronicity of her headaches, and my finding of a limited range of neck motion. Of course, the right shoulder stiffness was probably caused by the neck problem. [See my discussion elsewhere, for how to assess pectoralis major and minor tightness and shortening, but here is a hint – it has to do with the front of the armpit.]

20. So I would ask her to stand up and allow me to check her back. I would expose the back by lifting her shirt and (with her consent) opening her bra.

21. With my left arm I would put a hand around the front of her and palpate at least her right pectoralis muscle [front of the armpit] and then place my hand on her sternum to provide counter pressure while carefully palpating each medial-to-scapula soft tissue area and from low to high thoracic paraspinous soft tissue. It is very true that in both male and female patients this makes for some incidental contact with the breasts. [The issue of counterpressure is so important here. Any of you who have studied martial arts know that standing with your feet parallel is the weakest possible fighting stance. You can be knocked off balance by a front pressure of only 7 lbs, or a rear pressure of a mere 3 lbs! If you don't quickly learn this principle you will spend a lot of time on the mat.]

22. *If* I found a trigger point in the parascapular soft tissue, I would record it. *If* I found an increased soft tissue sense in the paraspinous soft tissue, I would attempt to reduce it with manual therapy – then I would record that: I didn't record these, so they weren't there [and so *I did no manual therapy on this lady* – remember Dr Bear had insisted that I make a record of what I had done, and I did. If it was not in the record, then it was not done].

23. In her complaint she says that I explained I "had to get closer" so squeezed between the bed and herself. [My object would be to get behind her and to her left.] These may indeed have been at close quarters – especially in the small cubicle area. My left antero-lateral [front, outer] thigh may indeed have made contact with her clothed [left] thigh or buttock – I have no idea that it did, because my attention was on my exam – but I have no reason to say that it couldn't have.

24. In this instance I found and recorded no further upper back pathology so would offer to fasten her bra. In my own office, my staff would spontaneously make this offer, to allow me to write in the chart.

25. She says I then proceeded to prescribe medication, and this is perhaps the only area of my real disagreement with her. In fact, I:

   a. *made a diagnosis* of mixed headache disorder;

   b. (to myself) *disapproved* of the Demerol, Gravol, and DHE treatment [because this appeared to be a fairly chronic problem, and Demerol only lasts about four hours];

   c. *Opted to treat her orally* insofar as she had not been throwing up [recently – the last had been at about 05:00 hrs, and it was now well after 15:00 hrs];

   d. *Wrote* an order at 15:47 for Valium 10 mg, Toradol 10 mg, Flexeril 20 mg, and Gravol 100 mg and may, in fact, have procured these from the med room and given them to her myself [I considered myself a staff member and would do what needed to be done, if no nurse were immediately at hand];

   e. *Arranged* for cervical (neck) x-rays, for XXXX [her family doctor] to be able to follow up with her; and,

   f. Had her remain in the area for 45 minutes to be sure she did not throw up the medication [that we had provided – by then the medications would be absorbing, and start to work].

26. I trust my approach worked on the headache and lasted longer than the Demerol/Gravol/DHE would have in a person who had had considerable exposure to narcotics in the past.

I trust this will explain the approach that I took. In my view, closeness certainly was a necessity in providing this assessment. Finally, unhooking the bra is something I do – with permission and with a female staff member present – every single day in medical practice and perhaps 5 or 6 times a day on busier days, Certainly every one of my office chaperones/staff members will be familiar with it. Every single time I obtain specific verbal permission – every single time, even as this complainant graciously concedes.

That was my response to a really vague complaint. I just said what I had done that day. Now I need to give you some idea of what her complaint became on the witness stand, perhaps informed by *the assuredly ethical* [might I seem sarcastic here too?] Counsel for the College that the nurse who had been in there would not be present to testify, so it would be her word against mine. It really is highly entertaining. On page 20 of the transcript, she pretty well rehearses back to us what she had said in her complaint letter. Fairly placid stuff – but vague. But then she adds new and interesting things – just read on, these are her *additional* words:

- Q: One hand or both hands on your breasts?
- A: Both hands
- Q: At the same time or do they alternate?
- A: Yes.
- Q: The same time?
- A: Yeah.
- Q: And you've described that his – and I think you said his bare arms are on the chest. Are the hands or the arms at all touching the nipple of your breasts?

- A: Yes.
- Q: And is it once or more than once that that occurs?
- A: More than once.
- Q: Now, you described Dr Litchfield's arms or hands on the front of your chest. Where are his hands pressing or touching?
- A: They were cupped over my breasts.
- Q: The fingers and the palm of the hands?
- A: Yes.
- Q: How long does this contact with the hands on your breasts take?
- A: Approximately, I would say, a minute or two. Less than two minutes.

[In fairness do you think any nurse on the planet would miss this clutch-from-behind move over a one or two minute time frame? No, I don't either. Well, except if that nurse were visually impaired and had a seeing-eye dog! Or perhaps, if the nurse had moved a table and chair into the curtained exam area so that she could catch up with charting.]

- Q: And I take it, it was not until you received medication at the hospital that these symptoms were relieved?
- A: I came home and I was still retching [Remember we'd had her stay in hospital for forty-five minutes to be sure that she didn't retch or throw up the pills. If she had, then we'd have had to use injection medications that can't be thrown up. In Europe, they usually use suppositories – I'm glad we didn't because that would be all the more fuel on the assault fire.] until the medication, the Gravol or whatever Dr Litchfield prescribed for me for the stomach upset, took effect.
- Q: And the migraine symptoms of this terrible headache? That also was present until the medication took effect.
- A: Right.

[So my treatment did work for her; it brought relief!]

She had distilled the encounter down to just a few short and sensational phrases, and my lawyer wanted to help her see that I had also collected some significant information in the history-taking portion of the assessment.

- Q: So when you say that the only thing that he asked you was how you were feeling, you're agreeing with me that there may have been large – or at least a number of further questions that he may have asked you that you don't recall at this point?
- A: That could be. I don't remember.

- Q: So you are saying that when Dr Litchfield examined you, he was behind you? [I and the nurse, after being "*miraculously found*" recalled that I did my examination from her left side.]
- A: Yes.
- Q: And the bed was between you and him?
- A: No, he slipped in behind – between me and the bed.

- Q: I understand you to say that you made eye contact with the nurse at that point?
- A: When he asked if he could undo my bra, I looked up at the nurse, and *we made eye contact* [this concession is so amazing because she conveniently has said that the nurse, who she expects won't be here to say otherwise, was distracted, not looking, or doing charts – just until the nurse's attention and focus become convenient to the telling of her tale, and only *then, they made eye contact!* So the nurse was at least attentive enough to make eye contact with her when she wanted her to – notice she didn't say that she had to throw a pillow at the nurse to catch her attention.] because I thought it was kind of an unusual question.

- Q: Now, Dr Litchfield undid the brassiere. Correct?
- A: Dr Litchfield –
- Q: Undid your bra.
- A: Yes, he did.

- Q: And I'm going to suggest that he put one hand around to the front of your body.
- A: No.
- Q: You are looking down to check the statement. Is that because you are not sure?
- A: Pardon me?
- Q: When I asked you that question, you looked down to check the statement. Is that because you're not sure?
- A: No. I am very sure.
- Q: I'm going to suggest that he felt in the region of your right shoulder, and then he placed his hand on the center of your chest or the sternum or the breastbone.
- A: No.
- Q: And he did, while he was examining you *check your back.* Correct?
- A: No.
- Q: *So you're saying at no time did he check your back?*
- A: *No.* [So now this witness, under oath, says that at no time did I check her back! But that is the whole foundation of allegation 7 – that to do a back assessment I asked permission and unclasped her bra; and also allegation 8 – that *in the examination of her back,* my assessment did not meet the standard because my left hand made contact with her bare breast! Here now, *she actually says there was no back exam!* So with this – her testimony under oath – there could not possibly be grounds to find me guilty of allegations 7 or 8!]
- Q: I'm going to suggest that he touched and pressed up and down your spine with one hand while he braced his other hand against the front of your chest.
- A: No.
- Q: And you said that he pressed against you, or he pressed you against him?
- A: He pulled me against him.
- Q: And you told the panel that you could feel his genitalia?
- A: Yes.

- Q: You could feel him pressing his genitalia against you or you against his genitalia?
- A: He pulled me against his body.
- Q: Well, his body or his genitalia?
- A: Well, his genitalia is part of his body. Right?
- Q: Did you feel his genitalia?
- A: Yes, I could.
- Q: Let's go to that page 82 [her statement]. Do you see that?
- A: M-hm.
- Q: Where *in there* [your statement] do you say that he was pressing you against his genitalia?
- A: Well, I said he was pulling me backwards until I could feel his body on my bum and legs.
- Q: Where in there do you talk about feeling his genitalia?
- A: Well, his body would be that . . . his body would . . . his body would . . . naturally that part of his body would fit my bum and legs. I mean, that part of his body would fit right there where my bum and legs are.
- Q: Where in the –
- A: Would it not?
- Q: Where in there do you talk about his genitalia?
- A: Well, that part of his body has his genitalia right there. Does it not?
- Q: Do you talk about being pressed against his genitalia in this statement?
- A: Well, that's part of his body. That's part of his anatomy.

Q: You don't say anything about his genitalia in that statement.

At this time the Counsel for the College feels the need to control things either as judge or as prosecutor and says, "I think the statement speaks for itself!" Is this the reason she was never interviewed by the investigator for the college? This really does sound like a judgment, doesn't it? Moreover, *why is he talking?* Does he understand that this witness is sabotaging his case and wants to prevent her?

- A: Well, I assume –

Again Counsel for the College: "You have asked the question three times, and she has given you her answer." Again, this sounds like the comment of a presiding judge. My lawyer resumes,

- Q: Well, in fairness, I don't believe that question has been answered.
- A: I mean, what am I supposed to . . . it's assumed. That part of his body fits right where my bum and legs are.
- Q: Now would you agree with me that Dr Litchfield is not a slim man. Fair?
- A: Is not a what?
- Q: He is not a slim man.
- A: Slim?
- Q: Yes.
- A: I have no idea. I have never really checked him out. Sorry. I don't know. I . . . I don't really . . . I don't really look at other men. I'm very happily married to one man.
- Q: I am going to suggest that if Dr Litchfield was standing behind you, it is the front of his body and his stomach that would be against you, not his supposed genitalia. [So I guess I'm grateful to have been overweight and to have attention drawn to that fact so well?!]
- A: When I bent over . . . I'm sorry, sir, I know what I felt.
- Q: You didn't write it.
- A: *Well give me a pen, and I will write it and initial it.*

[Surely there can't be a more obvious example of wanting to change evidence from what she said back then, to what she would like now to have said. This line, though, does make it clear that she did at some point provide a statement to someone and was familiar with the idea of changes being initialled or signed. So where is that statement? The defense never received a copy.]

- Q: You say when you bent over. What did you mean by that?
- A: I bent over from the waist.
- Q: How far did you bend?

- A: I don't know. Probably not . . . not in half for sure. Like, not very far.
- Q: Now, you have told us, I think, that he had both hands on your breasts.
- A: Yes.
- Q: You say that he touched your nipples?
- A: Yes.
- Q: Was that with his fingertips, with the palms of his hands, or what?
- A: That would be with the palms of his hands.
- Q: And you say that he had both hands on your chest for over a minute?
- A: I thought I said about a minute. [Remember she said one to two minutes. *It is so difficult to remember the exact lie that one tells!* Hence, the mismatch.]
- Q: About a minute.
- A: Yeah.
- Q: Were they moving or were they still?
- A: They were still for a while.
- Q: How long is a while?
- A: Fifteen seconds.
- Q: So he had both hands on your breasts, not moving for fifteen seconds.
- A: Yes.
- Q: With a nurse standing right there?
- A: Yes.
- Q: Watching what he was doing?
- A: No, she was charting or whatever.

[So again, she impugns the nurse for her lack of vigilance while I cupped each bare breast from behind, with *her bent forward* and *I* pressing my groin into her bum and legs, in front of that nurse! Is this complainant *"on drugs"*? (This reference to drugs, too, is from *My Cousin Vinny*, from the judge.) Her claim is sensational, wholly incriminating and completely fallacious, made-up.]

Then with regard to the close of the session, PF recalled the exam ending and, immediately after, she being given a prescription. However, an attempt was made to clarify her recollection by asking,

- Q: Well, in fact, what happened is that Dr Litchfield didn't say he was going to write a prescription. He told you you would have to have an x-ray. Correct?
- A: I can't remember. I don't remember that. It may have happened, but I don't remember it. [Well, that's convenient, isn't it?]
- Q: And in fact, you did have an x-ray that day.
- A: I can't remember that.
- Q: Before you had any medication prescribed for you, you had to go to the x-ray, and you had to have an x-ray done.
- A: That may have happened, but I don't remember it.

So there may be other things that happened, but she just "didn't remember." Now when the unfindable nurse was found, she denied that she had been charting in the room, and she denied the story of each hand cupping a breast at once. From page 267 lines 21 and 22, she felt confident that that didn't happen. Rather she describes one hand on the sternum as she believed, though she could not see it under PF's clothes, and the other hand palpating the back; certainly no "each hand cupping a bare breast" scenario. PF had talked extensively about my having pulled her backward into my body and genitals. From pages 268 and 269, this was simply denied also by this witness to the facts. Even after hearing Gaiana Brooker's evidence though, it was imperative for this prejudiced panel to dismiss it so that they could still be right in their condemnation. This, even though they were probably starting to become just a little bit uncomfortable. If uncomfortable, they did have, however, their *overwhelming moral certitude* about my overall guilt, probably because of Expert Witness 1's crusade. So they said of the nurse/chaperone's testimony: "The *recollection of the events by Ms Brooker LACKED some credibility* for the Panel in that she apparently could recall certain aspects of the visit in great detail, but had no recollection of *other significant aspects* of the visit." Oh really, members of the panel? And what were those *"significant" aspects* that she could not recall?

1. The *nature and style of clothes* PF had on. (page 276)
   [Now which of you panelists convinced the others that "any modern woman" would remember what clothing another lady wore five years previously? Was that you, Ms. Social Worker? I thought you were a feminist. The very idea of the overarching realm of fashion being easily remembered by any and all women is archaic and an insult to the women of today.]
2. *The patient seen just before PF.* (page 281)
   [It is true that for some unknown reason a recollection of this woman's examination remained in nurse Gaiana Brooker's mind while she seems to not remember the patient just before. However, might it be because Gaiana had a migraine disorder too, and this made her attentive? Maybe it was because while she acted as a chaperone for me she got to relax and observe *medicine being done, rather than having to do it,* and chart it, herself. Perhaps the patient just before this one didn't *need* a chaperone? Maybe it was a man or a child? I don't know why she remembers my exam of PF. But I know I am glad she was there, being observant, and did remember!]
3. *The manipulation of the back.* The chairman asked Gaiana, "Do you remember *what the manipulation looked like* in terms of can you describe this method of manipulation on that night?"

She responds, "I just recall him doing an examination of Ms F's back, and I can't really recall the manipulation."

"Aha," Dr. Chairman concludes to himself, "she can't even remember the manipulation that was done, yet she dares claim that she is sure nothing improper was done. How can she?" Wow, Chairman. I'm sure you're on the right track there. Crucify that villain Litchfield!

And then the social worker chips in, page 287 with the same question: "And as far as *the manipulation of the back*, what do you recall physically seeing?" To which Gaiana replies, "I don't!"

So why is it that a credible witness could not recall *"the manipulation"* of the thoracic spine? Come on, you know. Say it out loud – *because it wasn't done!* There was an assessment but no manual therapy. That is what I had *written*, that is what I had *said* in giving my evidence, and that is what the only other credible witness present (Gaiana Brooker) said. Committee, it was you who misunderstood. So don't fault Ms. Brooker for having a patchy memory. *There was no manipulation done – and she actually remembered that really quite clearly*, didn't she?

The thing that hurt the most about this was that the committee tried so desperately to prop up this lamentable complaint. They were willing to look foolish to do so. Over this willingness, I weep.

CHAPTER 6

MY EXPECTATION OF JUSTICE

LADY JUSTICE HAS been described, characterized, and sculpted many times over the years. Some of the imagery has her blindfolded. Others refute this idea because she has the pan balance in her (usually) left hand and a sword in her right hand. Those who deny the appropriateness of the blindfold tell us that she needs to see which evidence has tipped the scale – and she needs to see to effectively use the sword on the right person! So she may not be blind or blindfolded. Hence, the myth debunked that "justice is blind." She does carry the sword, with which to mete out the justice that is appropriate. No argument there. And she has in the other hand the pan-balance – a set of scales into one pan of which evidence is poured *against* the accused; into the other, evidence *for* the accused. Lady Justice does not personally influence the outcome. And that is the ideal – an impartial weighing of the evidence. As previously, I was scared of the complaints. I had been through this "meat grinder" before. I was anxious, often sleepless, and needed faith. Would things proceed fairly and completely? If so, I would again be exonerated. This is what I expected from my

College of Physicians and Surgeons: complete fairness. This would mean as follows:

1. Potentially biased administrators or panelists would recuse themselves (withdraw from the proceedings). For example, if an assistant registrar in charge of discipline recognized that in other college roles he had acquired personal knowledge of and an opinion about an accused, he would withdraw so that justice could be apparent and transparent.
2. A lawyer employed by the CMPA to defend me should at least consider recusing himself, if he had a personal and social relationship with the assistant registrar engaged in the disciplinary proceedings against me.
3. Expert witnesses called to testify for and against the accused physician (me) should be peers. This enables the comparison of physicians with similar background and training. This kind of expert witness can easily provide opinion about whether standards of care have not been met, have been met, or have been surpassed. A totally nonpeer expert witness makes for a remarkably difficult comparison and probably unfairness.
4. Witnesses who complain about a physician should be interviewed carefully and perhaps reinterviewed so that the exact complaint(s) can be identified, summarized, stated, and submitted to the defense. This allows a proper preparation of defense, or a clear statement that can be agreed with. This is called disclosure and is an element of common law. Imagine a situation in which you were ordered to come to court on such-and-such a date and only told on the stand what you were being accused of. It couldn't come close to fair, could it?
5. Once witness statements and statements by expert witnesses were received, they could not be changed. This has got to be a corollary to 4, above. The defense must know that which it must prepare to defend against: perhaps with other witnesses, perhaps with literature. Without it, there is a tilt in the scales of justice right from the start.

6. Lawyers or individuals acting without a lawyer must argue the case. This is just reasonable. Expert witnesses, specifically, provide evidence but do not argue the case. The service they are to provide is factual and correct information – or, when opinion, is declared as such. They can provide these opinions, but it isn't "their case" to argue.

7. Expert witnesses would not proffer evidence from one source that would tend to condemn and *exclude evidence from that same source that would tend to exculpate* (exonerate) *the accused.* That would show expert witness bias and surely tip the scales, of course.

8. Expert witnesses would refrain from proffering information beyond their area of expertise, as no one is an expert in all things. If an opinion is outside their area of training, they would comfortably disclose that fact.

9. Judges, or panels of judges, would not be biased or partial. Years ago, there was a very famous feud between two American families: the affluent Hatfields of West Virginia and the less wealthy McCoys of Kentucky. This is possibly the best known feud between real people, in the world. Only Shakespeare's *Romeo and Juliet* with its feuding Capulet and Montague families has been more studied. No Capulet would want a Montague judge, and no McCoy would feel safe in the hands of a Judge Hatfield. The impartiality and fairness of the judge is certainly the cornerstone of justice.

10. Judges would be honest and accurate.

11. Even if judges had what they considered to be a personal knowledge of medicine, they would not *inject their "own knowledge" into the proceedings without the defense having a chance to prepare for the additional "evidence."* Such would again create "an uneven playing surface" – the favoring of one party over the other.

12. Lawyers would be honest with each other and to the judge. Perhaps I am being naive here. Perhaps they lie to each other constantly.

13. The roles of each person in the system would be well defined so that the responsibilities and parts each play are very clear – and all would know how to interface with the players.

Of course, I would want my own lawyer to work well with me. Legal proceedings of any significance tend to be very expensive. In view of this, I did what virtually every physician in the country does, by regularly paying litigation insurance to the Canadian Medical Protective Association. Then, should any accusation arise, legal fees are then paid by the insurance organization. But they contract with a specific law firm in each province in Canada. "Contracted lawyers" get lots of volume and tend to not challenge the way that the college does its legal business, including an *"our lawyer also gets to be the administrative judge"* thing. They just learn to know what to expect. So what happens when one lawyer in the province gets all the CMPA's sexual impropriety cases, and you're charged with something akin to that [and I really pray it won't happen to you]? Well then, you've just got to get along with him. 'Cause he's the guy! You might find him hard to understand. You might feel that you can't make yourself understood by him. You might feel him to be already prejudiced about you. You may find he doesn't ask you enough pertinent questions to allow your full participation in your own defense. You may hear him, in presenting your direct evidence, question *where you had learned* to ask the screening question of a female patient, "Are you able to orgasm (from a CME course in Saskatoon – to allow her the opportunity to raise any concerns in that area)?" And then when presenting your technique of breast examination, that included attempting to express any secretions present from the nipple, *fail to ask you from where you had learned that technique* (a pivotal error)! You may think he dismisses any suggestions that you do make. You may find that he creates his whole defense with very little input from you, assuming that he just "knows best." You may discover that he has chosen a junior lawyer of your faith from his firm to mollify you. You may feel that he is not tearing off his metaphoric coat to stick on a pole and wave the banner: "This man is innocent!" You may find that he is asking you to *plead guilty* "to some of the lesser charges" without being aware that pleading guilty is the start of a very slippery slope. You may ask that junior cocounsel whether you can trust him and hear a vague, politically correct answer about not being able to comment on her supervising lawyer. You may confront him with your unhappiness at his efforts in your behalf. You may hear him <u>fail</u> to ethically review your legal options at that point! You may really want another lawyer because you've been privileged to see law practiced with honor, critical thinking, and strength. You may ask CMPA to let you have a different lawyer. You know what? CMPA will say that it is "certainly your right to seek a lawyer whom YOU would then pay" [and it will be very, very costly]. Otherwise rely on our (the CMPA's) choice! Eventually, the CMPA did allow me to change lawyers. But by then, *the findings had been written, and they could not be altered.*

It is hard enough to face the profound criticism of a disciplinary hearing. Your lawyer has to be on your side. And I have listed for you the thirteen expectations I had of procedural fairness. At stake was my livelihood and professional standing. I believed that I had committed my life to the most ethical of professions and therefore awaited the demonstration of each of these thirteen characteristics. What are the chances, statistically, that one of them would not be in place? What about two or up to five not being in place? What about all thirteen? To have none of them in place would be a great disappointment, indeed! It would make anyone feel conspired against. What did happen?

Item 1:

My initial lawyer interacted with the assistant registrar, who discussed the issues in turn with the college chairman of the complaints committee. Then this chairman of the complaints committee became the assistant registrar in charge of complaints. And next, he became the registrar. All the while, he was directly involved with the final four complainants against me.

We understand that voting in the U.S. Congress and the U.S. Senate is often preeclipsed by the garnering of votes by personal commitment to a lobbyist or organizer. (My wife loved the movies *Legally Blond.*) Would it not be naïve to think that this never happened in colleges of physicians and surgeons? When you sit and have a casual conversation with the registrar over coffee or with a beer after curling, do you not think he might have a personal agenda for your friendly meeting? Might he be seeking your personal commitment on an issue? But he would probably like you the better if you would kindly not allow yourself to consider ulterior motives! If ever there was a good definition of networking, it would be in this forum. It used to be called the old boys' system. This comes from a history in the private schools where there would be new boys, old boys, and a head boy. The head boy held a lot of power. He could make your years a living hell. His kind of "bullying" was never in check. Hmm!

Item 2:

Right from the start, my assigned lawyer had told me that he was a personal friend to that assistant registrar for the college – the one who dealt directly with me. That at least made a *potential* conflict of interests. But of course, some lawyers wouldn't let that influence them. I should just take it on faith that he was one of those, right? I wonder if he would want his CMPA client to know that I directly questioned his commitment to help me while his junior cocounsel sat there – months before the hearing occurred – and he failed to ethically review the legal alternatives available to me. Would he want his CMPA client to know that he bluntly *slammed* me with the final decision: "You'll never be able to practice medicine anywhere in the civilized world; ever!" Lawyers seem to choose their words pretty carefully. Why did he choose those words? Do you agree that the words seem to convey some hostility? But of course, he was not being hostile with his CMPA *client*, only with me – *the accused physician*.

Item 3:

The chairman of the committee asks me questions with an obvious bias:

1. *"If you actually thought* that a patient might think you are coming onto them by examining their nipples in that fashion prior to or as you are examining them, wouldn't you think it

prudent to say 'I need to do this for this reason,' just because it's a sensitive issue?" (page 634). I gave my answer that *I hadn't thought that* a patient might think I am coming onto them by examining their nipples in that fashion, at all. But notice the question. It is so very biased. Is it meant to trap me? Is it rhetorical (not to be answered), or is it asked to create stress? What the committee member was referring to was that when JM asked about the exam that had been done some months previously, I showed her the Novey textbook with my explanation.

Burt Lancaster had a role in the movie *Field of Dreams*. He played a retired doctor who says to Kevin Costner that he has to get home to his wife so that "she doesn't get to thinkin' I've got a girl friend." It was in that same spirit that I said to JM that "I wouldn't want her to get to thinkin' that I was coming on to her" when she specifically questioned why I had examined her using nipple expression, while I showed her one textbook that specifically demonstrated with pictures that we should proceed this way.

2. "Do you have any literature to support the necessity of breast milk expression as a diagnostic measure for – diagnostic for breast cancer?" Wow, what a question! No time to prepare in defense for such a thing. If there were such literature, I had no forewarning it would be called for. Of course, as you have read, the point of expressing the breast in a lactating mother with a red nipple is to check for duct occlusion or expressible pus.

3. "What would be the purpose of running your fingers from her (exposed) chest, in short, rapid motions down to her pubic area?" Now, to me, this sounds sort of like part of a piano performance, but I guess at this point they had judged my guilt, and so did not really weigh the concocted complaint phrases very carefully. My answer, of course, was "None. That did not happen!"

4. "Do you think that in a girl age 20 or a woman under 30, that the incidence of actually finding malignant cells (on the cytology slide that you prepare) is actually significant?" This, of course, refers to the Dunn method published in 1995, in the *British Journal of Surgery*. To this question, my answer is that if the cells are there, I want to know about it.

On page 629, line 17, the transcripts show that I stated that there were "two things" that could be gleaned from doing nipple expression as a part of breast exam. I focused on the first one and explained it. The chairman summarized the "first thing" by saying, "So the only benefit that you're getting for the patient's benefit (in that situation) is to show that you can express secretions, and that they are OK?" And I agreed to that, for those (the first thing) that have physiological discharge (secretions). Unfortunately for the clarity of the proceedings, he never did get me to elaborate the *"second thing": to ascertain whether the expressed secretions are pathological.* The transcript doesn't show enlightenment to be this chairman's purpose. He was *there to condemn and mock me.*

My own lawyer asked that I clarify why I would (as I always did on every female patient) attempt to express secretions on PV who was still breast-feeding. I responded that you might discover TWO things. I then went on to elaborate *the first* of the two things. First, the discovery of *complete* duct obstruction witnessed by a "white bleb" (which is epithelialization, with milk behind it, over a blocked duct) or tangential streaming of milk (coming from *partial* epithelialization) from a duct in the process of blocking. I further explained the treatment of these issues. Unfortunately, my lawyer carried on the questions in another direction before I gave *the second* thing: that might be discovered from the expression of the breast ducts in a breast-feeding woman who, in this case, had a little nipple redness. That is, frank pus coming from one of the ducts. This would identify the *adenitis* (not cellulitis) form of mastitis and need to be treated with an antibiotic.

Item 4:

Witness PF was never interviewed after sending in her original brief and vague letter of complaint. This did not allow the defense to prepare a defense. The playing field tilts further. Why?

Item 5:

Dr. DDDD's opinion was sought in the prehearing correspondence with the college. I was sent copies of the expert witness statements that had been received. She wrote, and I quote: "*Older methods* of clinical breast examination *DO suggest* that the nipples be checked for discharge but this practice has been largely abandoned, as it serves no useful purpose." This is pretty forthright, isn't it? She thought my actions were outdated, but she had heard of them being done. So at worst, I was being charged with being outdated! But then in the hearing *SHE CHANGED this testimony*, and when questioned under oath about the change said, "When I first wrote this, *I was giving him the benefit of the doubt* . . ." (page 325). What does this "benefit of the doubt" mean? Either she was aware of this being an older examination technique, or she wasn't. She didn't say, "I gave him the benefit of the doubt by accepting that *if he said* he had learned that technique from a reputable source, *then he had*." No! So it couldn't be called a benefit of the doubt, coming from the largess of her soul that caused her to allow that nipple expression in the course of a routine breast exam might be an older technique, and therefore legitimate. (I guess that is why lawyers ask for an explanation of why a previous statement differs from what is said on the witness stand.) She knew it as a technique! But she *decided to claim otherwise under oath*, during the hearing. *Which was untrue*: the former or the latter? Had she simply come to the hearing as an expert witness who completely lacked impartiality, honesty, or fairness – OR was she doing a favor for someone? Did you just do what your old mentor asked, Mde l'Expert? This reminds us of George Orwell's *1984*, in which the then-government would change the states against whom they warred and then, with new alliances and new enemies, claim that the way they had changed things was the way it had always been. And the people were expected to simply accept the blatant lie. In this case she has provided evidence that it was an older technique, and then maintains that it was never a technique. Does this also qualify as a blatant lie? Certainly, *panel members seeking to discern truth* would at least have some misgivings about the integrity of this *expert witness*, if that discernment was *at some point* their goal.

Items 6 and 7:

As discussed, expert witness 1 for the college either did not receive any understanding of her role as an expert, or chose to set it aside and approached the case with a chosen side which she wanted to make win. Expert 1 also forwarded to the college (and hence, the defense) her view that examination of the breast that included an attempt to express nipple secretions was outdated and then, under oath, changed that stance to one that said that it was never recommended – allowing the defense no chance to prepare a defense for that revised premise. Further, the expert *raised from* among family practice literature evidence that she could bend to seem against me, and *excluded* from the same article evidence that upheld my approach.

Item 8:

As discussed, college expert 1 pretends also to be an expert in breast-feeding medicine and infections during lactation, although she has no credentials in these and shows herself incorrect in what she did assert.

Items 9 and 10:
THE COMMITTEE WITHHOLDS AND EMBELLISHES

The committee, as I said, felt the need to go *further* than the evidence. They referred to it once on page 4 of their findings, three times on page 7, twice on page 8, and once on page 9 as "REMOVING" rather than "unclasping" her brassiere. That is *seven times*! Why did they substitute the phrase "removing the brassiere," for undoing or unclasping the bra? Might it be because it sounds more assaultive and violent than unclasping? What do you think? If you are going to do violence against a doctor, is it important to suggest that *his behavior was violent?* Then anything done to him can seem justified! The CBC Radio 1 in February 2010 aired a radio program called *Ideas* to deal with the premise "Some of the greatest *atrocities* are committed by those who have *overwhelming moral certitude* . . . and then they are often found wrong." So what do you think, committee, did your foregone "overwhelming moral certitude" come from expert 1's crusade? Did that make it okay to keep referring to the unclasping of a bra as "removing a bra"? You certainly *made it sound* like violence against women. The facts don't really matter here, do they? Because you had your *overwhelming moral certitude*, right? Is that also called situational ethics or just a *lack of ethics?* The public definitely knows the buzz phrase "violence against women." If you make my actions sound violent, then it's all right whatever happens to me and my family, right? Ms. Social Worker, I think you have given new meaning to the title of your job – the worker of social wrath! It's the harm you can justifiably cause socially 'cause you were so certain of your rightness and that of expert 1, right?

The committee found that "an admitted pattern of practice which invades the privacy, touches women's breasts in what can only be construed as unnecessary and inappropriate – *damages the integrity of the profession* as one which should act only in the patient's best interest. His conduct is found to be unbecoming of a Physician."

Remember that it was at least one member of the committee who read the article by Monica Morrow and quoted from it while failing to acknowledge the words that were part of the same sentence, which would have confirmed my method of physical examination. So who really has damaged the integrity of our professions, committee members?

Item 11: The committee adds its own evidence

There is no built-in protection against evidence being introduced by the doctors on the committee: that renders the teams uneven. Three glaring examples of these assumptions in this particular hearing are

1. that the committee made the mistaken assumption that my reference to screening for costochondritis as a part of my upright assessment of the thoracic spine, was not normal parlance and therefore suspicious;
2. that to check the tone of the pectoralis major and minor, a woman's breast was likely to be fondled rather than this assessment being done from the front of the armpit; and
3. that they understood the Durrani and Winnie reference, and that it meant that a physician should focus on greatly relaxing his patient so that the piriformis muscle could be directly palpated vaginally and, much more dangerously, rectally! That the piriformis syndrome has "nothing to do with the pubo – and other coccygeus muscles."

When the panelists hearing the evidence can add evidence of their own that is not subject to anticipation, preparation, evaluation, and defense – again, there is intrinsic unfairness added to the proceedings. Moreover, their "additions to the evidence" were incorrect, in each of these instances.

Item 12: The lawyer who judges other lawyers

With a new legal team we sought a judicial review. Counsel for the college stridently maintained, and the judge eventually agreed, that the application for judicial intervention was PREMATURE, with the expectation that the college *could* correct its errors. Of course, Counsel for the College did let on to His Honor that *the findings reached by the committee in error could never be altered.* He withheld that from the bench. But then, after new evidence was heard by the committee, he was very quick to remind *its members* that they were *NOT ABLE to change or modify their findings!* Why such a quick reminder? Perhaps he saw that the evidence that had then been heard was really strongly in my favor. My new and excellent lawyers, Dana Schindelka and Deanna Steblyk [I just had to use their names because they comported themselves with dignity, honor, and strength] could not stop the avalanche that followed.

There are probably some of you who live quiet suburban lives, honestly believing pretty well everything that you read in the paper or see on TV. Most of you may figure that if it has been through some hearing process or trial, and has been decided, then *those conclusions have just got to be accurate, right?* Because that is the simplest way to think about it, right? Somebody else has supplied you a conclusion, and so you don't have to think about or ponder it. If you really believe that, then set this book right down. To read it and understand how these errors were made takes analytical thinking. It's no shame to say you don't have that skill. And the world will continue to seem a very predictable, reliable place . . . unless you are ever charged with something YOU didn't do. Will you then figure it'll be the first time, in the history of mankind that that has EVER happened?

The falseness came right from the start. Official transcript, page 13: (My former lawyer) "At this time, I do not anticipate that you will be hearing from *any* of the chaperones: either because we cannot identify the person who is present, or because the person who was present has no specific recollection of the events, and that applies not just to Dr Litchfield's office, but it applies to the hospital, where there were times when there was a nurse present, as you will hear, but either the hospital can't identify the nurse, or whoever was present has no recollection of the events in question. *I understand that is correct, (college counsel)?*" It is so important that you understand that my lawyer is *deferring to college counsel* for the answer to this question. As a fellow lawyer admitted to the bar these lawyers are sworn, as officers of the court, to be honest with the bench and with each other. They are "on the record." They have communicated prior to the hearing and my lawyer trusts in the college counsel's word. *And Counsel for the College says, "Yes."* This is after the college has done its' "investigation," of course.

The disciplinary committee in their *penalty* portion finally had only *begun* to see the light (page 289). The chairman says after listening to the "lost, now found" nurse who attended the examination of PF: "I have one question to (Counsel), *as a representative of the College.* When I look at this record, I see the signature of Ms. Brooker at the bottom right-hand corner of the nurse's section. IT JUST LOOKS SO CLEAR TO ME, and I am just wondering why we (YOU) missed this before?"

And the Counsel for the College says, "I HAVE NO ANSWER."

The chairman continues, "Because *even myself*, when I remember looking at this record prior, I thought I recognized or remembered from before that WE COULD NOT IDENTIFY . . . [the identity of the nurse chaperone]!"

So that's it, counsel? *Your answer is that you have no answer?* Are we to, then, chalk it all up to the excellent proficiency of the "investigative" part of the college organization, or *was the witness intentionally unfound?* Your having no answers worries pretty well everyone reading this book, that you actually may *have* some answers. Go on, guess at an answer. The chairman of the disciplinary committee who got the wrong findings is asking you a question. Do you have no answer to *articulate* because there are some secrets here? Remember how the counsel for the defense relied on you for her *unfindability?* And he trusted you as a lawyer admitted to the bar to give an honest answer. And you confirmed that she was unable to be found? Have you broken your oath to the bar?

Item 13:

College traditions have evolved to the point that the prosecuting attorney ALSO MUST ACT as legal advisor to the college *AND* consider himself senior legal authority at the hearing. Maybe it started with regular lawyer stuff like, "I object to this question, Mr Chairman." Following which, the chairman sustains the objection of Counsel for the College. When you've played the tape enough, and the Counsel for the College's objections have never been unsustained, perhaps he stops even involving the chairman, kind of like a JUDGE himself, interrupting or cutting off whenever he feels like it, because this is the tradition that has evolved. That makes three roles by the one person. Virtually every defending lawyer will be frustrated by this, but if they are frequently defending at the college, they won't try to buck the system: *they will have come to expect it.* Only lawyers unfamiliar with the "college way" will really be surprised and struggle against this embedded wrongness. For example, generally my first lawyer pretty well let the Counsel for the College run the show. However, in the second (or penalty) portion of my disciplinary hearing, I was armed with two "new lawyers." One of them was leading evidence from the nurse that the college had been unable to find, but who had been imminently findable. She asked the nurse, "Do you believe you would have been able to tell if he was doing any of those things, given that his hands were underneath her clothes?" Now here the lawyer for the college, trying to wear three different hats, interjects, "Well, that's a hypothetical question." My lawyer starts to say, "I'm asking for her . . ." when he cuts her off again with, "Well, she's not here to give you an opinion on what she believes she could have done. She can recall, and she can say what she saw or didn't see, but it is not an appropriate question to ask a lay witness what they believe could have happened." My lawyer then cooperates by saying, "Allow me to rephrase it. Ms. Brooker, you mentioned that in fact from your position, standing in front of the patient, you mentioned that you did not see his hands move (one in front and one behind the patient) . . ." to which the nurse agrees. Then further along in the proceedings, this gem (official transcripts, penalty portion of disciplinary hearing, page 270): "Have you ever seen him do anything that you considered to be inappropriate with a female patient?" And in chimes the college lawyer again (acting as judge, to which he has become very used): "Well, you can ask her questions about the patient she is here to testify about. She is not here to give evidence about standards. She is only here to say what she saw or didn't see. She is not an expert." Now here of course, college counsel is on quicksand. This is a very experienced nurse, and really *she is an expert* observer! (See the chapter on PF, later in the text.) My lawyer resumes, "Exactly! And I am asking her for what she saw." The college counsel doesn't like this kind of commentary on the record, so he says, "With this patient that's fine." [This is his final adjudication, *AS JUDGE*! Perhaps the college should have given him a gavel to hold for these moments.] However, as one of my new lawyers, Deanna Steblyk, won't be cowed by him. She states, "The actual question as to what she has seen with respect to his conduct with female patients that she has witnessed *and* the facts in question."

Here, Mr. College Counsel knows he's losing ground despite the pompousness that all these roles impose on him. He says now in his judge role, "You have asked her about appropriateness, and that is a standard." Now, are you ready for this? Deanna confronts him, *the guy who thinks he is a judge*! (Page 270 of penalty transcripts): "GIVEN that *you don't make rulings on objections*, perhaps the committee could give us some direction."

So here, the chairman of the committee is *obliged to actually chair* something, but he does want to prop up the obviously wrong college counsel. So he says, "Well, I appreciate the comments of Mr (BBB) with regards to the *standards that he has raised* [lol] or the question over standards, and I think you should rephrase your question." So he seems to be propping up the "judge/prosecutor/advisor," but then he says, "But I don't mind you asking the witness what she has seen in past events working with Dr. Litchfield." Uh-oh, Mr. BBB, *the actual judges are allowing that evidence*! You must feel soooo bad! Deanna asks, "Ms. Brooker, have you ever seen anything in past instances working with Dr Litchfield while he has been examining female patients, have you ever seen anything that gave you cause for concern?" To this the nurse answers, "No." Deanna continues, "As someone who worked with Dr Litchfield for a number of years, can you provide the committee with your overall impression of Dr Litchfield?" And Nurse Brooker kindly says of me, "I believe that Dr Litchfield was a very competent physician and was definitely an asset to the XXXX Hospital, you know being a rural hospital in a small community. And I would think he was one of the best doctors we had in XXXX."

So then, what if the powers in a college are not divided? What if the registrar maintains control of the employment of the legal counsel (*and IMPOSES his triple role*), and the influence from the registrar or assistant registrar also controls the preset notions and proceedings of the hearing, and therefore, so much of the outcome? Could the registrar thrive . . . even as a bully?

In a letter to Bishop Mandell Creighton in 1887, Lord Acton is quoted as saying: "Power tends to corrupt, and absolute power corrupts absolutely. Great men are almost always bad men." Maybe that should read, "Very powerful men are almost always bad men" because the powerful aren't necessarily "great." And there are powerful men who truly are great.

As it turns out, the college produced only one of the chaperones (HH, witness to WG) as a material witness because the college counsel felt she did his case some good. But neither the college nor my then legal counsel "finds" any of the other three chaperones. My wife, Dianne, can't remember the encounter with PV but (unfortunately for the college counsel) PV can remember that it was my wife whom I called into the room in the midst of the counseling appointment during which I reduced a somatic dysfunction of her midback, and so my wife became a rebuttal witness. The college lawyer had pretty well rehearsed with PV to say that I had placed a hand on each of *her breasts at the same time*, like PF had claimed. Now, that allowed Dianne to give her rebuttal evidence, and she said that she had never seen any such maneuver (one hand on each breast from behind at the same time) in any clinical situation, and therefore it did not happen in front of her with PV, either. Despite all of the counsel's best challenges, she never did relent: "No, Counsel, the two hand thing never did happen, even if I can't recall this specific exam! *It didn't ever happen to any patient* that I saw my husband assessing or treating!" [Remember, my kids had figured she was the more assertive of the two of their parents! Counsel, Counsel, you picked the wrong Momma to mess with.] And that meant that there were *actually three out of four of the principal chaperones found*; none of them independently confirming any breast fondling! Ouch! The house of cards is a-comin' down!

Of course, to me, the allegation was painful, and the college's handling of the allegations was distinctly anguishing from a group who represented the governance of the profession that I had given so much of my life to. The take-home message for you is to not let your title or position define you, so that if you lose that title or position, *you have lost yourself.* I hadn't had this insight during the proceedings, and this made me the more vulnerable: I made myself responsible for what clearly was due to an unlevel balance in the justice that was applied to me. I really did feel defeated and that I had not defended myself adequately – the consequence of which was that I could not provide for my wife and family! There were deep aches here that I see caused some posttraumatic stress. I survived because Dianne (mainly) held my head above water while the torrents came on. My religious services and my home observance of prayer and scriptural meditation helped. The books on my night table helped: Victor Frankl and Jesus Christ, two Jews – one a survivor, the other a divine martyr. My children helped so much, although many of them don't know all of the details here. I didn't have a puppy then, but that too is a helpful relationship; she occupies time and adores each family member even if she's not yet completely obedient. Maybe total obedience was never what I was seeking in a pet, and I hear she is doing better.

Abe Maslow brought forward his "pyramid of needs" from the foundation of survival, security, social, self-reliance, and on to the pinnacle of self-actualization. For social needs, we have only spouse, family, friends, work, and religion – and I'm adding pets. When one of these is threatened, we only have the others to help us maintain social stability. If social stability falters, then security and perhaps survival can become threatened.

THE ONE WITNESS THAT THE COLLEGE "COULD" FIND

Counsel for the College liked having Hazel as a witness. With his "ethical legal guidance," she says about my providing an explanation to the patient before doing an exam or manual therapy:

I don't *recall* him giving any explanation (page 153, line 7);

- There was *very little* explanation (same page, line 11) [inferring, "but, now I recall . . . there was very little"];
- Now, Counsel for the College is probing to see how malleable this witness might be [what he can get her to say], so he then asks, "And that would be before the vaginal examination occurred, there was *NO* explanation given?" To which Hazel answers, "M-hm." And he confirms, "Is that yes?" So he has taken her from "I don't recall the explanation" to "very little

explanation," to "*no* explanation given." Cool. I'll bet no one even noticed, Counsel.

- He goes on, "And before . . . the manual therapy, there was *no explanation* given?" To which Hazel replies, "Not to my knowledge, no. Not that I recall." What might have diminished her recall about dialogue between the doctor and this very chatty patient? Could it have been that very thing: the chattiness?
- That was on page 153 of the transcript. Then on page 169, *during the cross-examination of this same witness*, my lawyer asks, "Now, you indicated that Dr Litchfield did some manual therapy or manipulations on her at the end of the examination. Is that right?" "Yes," she says. My lawyer continues, "And *he explained* to her where or how to move to do these?" To which she answers, "Yes." So this witness actually DOES recall *some explanations* although, just moments before, the Counsel for the College got her to say that there had been "no explanation" at that time.
- And what she further recalls is, "Mrs XXX tends to talk the whole time, and that's not unusual for her, in my experience." Page 153 and also page 154: "She kind of just keeps talking." Can you conceive of an explanation being given and, with the patient chattering, the nurse not actually registering the explanation? Perhaps *even the chatterer* did not understand that an explanation was given. But at some point, the chatterer's purpose became to seek a nice fat settlement cheque!

MAKING MONEY FROM LAWSUITS

"Dr Litchfield," you're bound to ask, "how can you state so firmly that this patient was going for money? How could you possibly know that this particular lady actually went out looking for opportunities to *sue and profit from law suits?*" That is a very good question. You're thinking clearly. Well, of course, she did sue me. And as it turns out, ongoing legal suits are very much her "thing"; actually they are *a matter of public record* in Canada. I am one of seven people sued by this patient. Two of them curiously involve injuries sustained from falling off faulty toilet seats at very successful franchised fast food outlets. Two of them! Wow! Clearly these businesses have money, and this lady knows how to become enriched from the "accidents" and "encounters" that she has had. Think to yourself how many times you've been injured in a fall from a toilet seat. None? Do you know of *anyone* who has been so injured? Yeah, I'm a doctor of family medicine and emergency, and I *never* have treated anyone in my twenty-six years of practice for that type of injury. I think you could assume, though, that if a person *had ever been* so injured, he/she would be bloody sure the public toilet seat was sound before using it! It can't take more than a few seconds. Doesn't pretty well *everyone in the civilized world* briefly check out an unknown toilet seat before sitting on it? This lady wants you to believe that after one significant injury, she still didn't! This lady made a claim and got a settlement for her injury in one instance and is currently pressing another. Wow!

On the other hand, she had already talked with her lawyer before she typed out her outlandish complaint letter to the college (but never the police – doesn't that tell you something?). She was seen by me in the wee hours of Sunday, the thirtieth of December 2001. She crafted her letter of complaint by Tuesday, the second of January 2002: the day after New Year's Day. And she's already conferred with her lawyer! She was calculating and crafting her letter within three days. Her lawyer certainly might remember the accusations that had previously been levelled against me. Her lawyer may well have informed her that I was this *horrible predator* who had never previously been stopped. He may have envied the profound skills of my previous well-known lawyer. He may have wanted to challenge his own metaphoric Goliath.

On a more subtle level, she knew that I did manual therapy. Sometime well previously, I had assessed her for migraine headache, and she had an associated neck problem, which I call cervical somatic dysfunction. I did manual therapy on her neck and her migraine disappeared, virtually immediately. No drugs were required. I had clearly helped her. But after having received manual therapy, the muscles often attempt to tighten back up and pull the problematic segment back out of alignment, hence the need to use heat and possibly muscle relaxants after treatment, which she may or may not have done. Well, I noted in my office notes related to this woman that she had called my office in the city nineteen days later and complained of my treatment, saying that a few days later her neck had become very stiff. She wanted me to *undo what I had done.* I offered to see her at my office or on the next trip that I made out to that rural hospital, but she never showed. So I am left to wondering, did she fabricate some of the situation which I faced with her on the thirtieth of December 2001 before being seen? She certainly could not have forgotten that I do manual therapy. Not after she had made a previous complaint to me about it.

Each time that I saw her I had done my best to help. It was hurtful to hear her diminish what I had considered to have been an elaborate attempt to help that required all of my special training – above and beyond average management. She simply wasn't the least bit grateful for the assistance and rewrote history to conform with the media suspicion from 1989 so that she could also sue the medical authority for their having allowed me to practice in an emergency room setting in spite of all of the previous complaints made SO public. Her lack of gratitude for help was not unique, of course, in medicine.

DRUG SEEKING

A further issue with this lady is the question of drug seeking. The fine committee stated on page 22 of their findings in my regard that "he attempted to discredit Ms WG by stating that she may have been drug seeking *based on her comment* that 'I'm not sure why I'm here, cause you can't fix a tailbone.'" Interesting summary, committee, but NO! I didn't base my concern about drug seeking on that comment. Rather, I based my view on these facts:

- That she had Fiorinal at home (from her complaint letter).
- That she had been popping Percocet all day (from the nurse who answered her phone calls at the hospital).

- That she proffered that her regular doctor had told her that if the *pain* got bad then she was to "go to the hospital and get a *shot*" (from her letter of complaint).
- That in her complaint letter of 145 lines, 43 lines (=29.7%) are dedicated to seeking a shot of narcotic that was not provided, and telling us that (in spite of the profound nausea and vomiting that she was experiencing) she was not able to improve until she accessed some *oral* Demerol and Gravol through illegal sources – unauthorized family members [but wait, if she was nauseated and vomiting, how did she manage to keep down those oral medications?].
- That she felt that "*all of this could have been avoided had Dr Litchfield simply acted in accordance with the immediate problem*, e.g. the migraine and the vomiting. I worked all New Year's Eve day 'hung over' from the drugs and was too sick to join my family (children) on New Year's Eve." All of this could have been avoided had Dr Litchfield simply *acted in accordance with the immediate problem*? Huh! What did you say? That's not what a sexually assaulted person would say when she does complain!

What is the translation of what she's just said? This would have never happened if Dr Litchfield had just given me the drugs (narcotic injection) that I wanted. So she is telling us that the thing that bugged her the MOST, is that she didn't get her drugs. It's really quite revealing, isn't it? When lying, a person so often can't knit together all the pieces of the story that they provide to support that lie.

This woman complained that contrary to what the nurse and I said about our entering the room together, I had – according to her – gone in ahead of the nurse and groped her right breast by reaching up under her hospital gown [which would have been a *clear* sexual assault].

So she tries to give this encounter the taint of sexual assault right from the start: an aggression against women. She says she has been violated! What should we expect her to say, then, in this portion of the complaint letter? Let's take a whack at it. So I'll be her: "*All of this could have been avoided if Dr Litchfield weren't such a damned pervert!"* [Please forgive this swear. I was trying to be in character for someone else, not me.] See! Doesn't that sound more like someone who has been assaulted? What she says, instead, focuses on the drugs for which she had to seek from unauthorized sources: her "entitlement," even if she had presented with back pain radiating down the right leg. She still deserved a shot for pain, just like she'd have gotten for a migraine! Right?

CHAPTER 7

BEFORE AND AFTER THE COMMITTEE REPORTED TO COUNCIL

THIS COMMITTEE PRO-DUCED its scathing set of findings following the hearing in 2005. These would then be used as a springboard for the penalty portion of the hearing with the same fine folk. It is very hard to describe how unfairly I felt I had been treated. Awkward, too, because *I was not sure I had done my best* at getting my lawyer to effectively represent me. That is, that I brought this upon myself – *just the way so many rape victims feel.* I was in a spin. Despite the love that I had for the Christian religion that I was a part of, I was again being accused of unfaithfulness to my dear wife. Could she withstand it? Was she able to hold her head upright in public? I was terrified – not really for myself, but for those who so clearly depended on me! I was constantly ruminating over things I ought to have done. I was overtly anxious to drive past my former lawyer's building or the building where the college had its offices. I was anxious on my way to work. My essential tremor became much more significant. I was noted by my staff to have elevated blood pressure. Did I say before how my office staff were *the best*?

As the college investigator had dug around among the nurses out in XXXX, she found one nurse, yet had missed finding Gaiana Brooker. She found this nurse had been uncomfortable with the recollection of one of my in-city patients whom I had asked to come out to XXXX when she had a problem. I don't even know who it was. Was it you, HH? Is that why the college figures you where "their" witness? This young patient had previously been my receptionist, and I had attended her in two pregnancies. I loved watching her and her husband grow as parents and those two dear little children grow in their home. I really felt the bliss of family practice right there: watching the families grow. DV was a pretty lady. Her husband was a rugged, humorous, and thoughtful skilled worker. They were "good people" but not rich. Their times of having children were over, but they blossomed in other ways. DV worked hard at losing to her the distressed image of "Yah, I'm just a mom." She exercised every day. Muscles grew stronger. She became healthier. I arranged for her to see a plastic surgeon to have a breast reduction. It was a bit complicated, but I managed those complications for the plastic surgeon. We family doctors do that so often for the "specialists." She got hematomas and seromas, and I just dealt with them because they were familiar to me. Probably while I still had DV as my receptionist, I had removed an almost two kilogram lipoma from an abdominal wall, after first ensuring by CT scan that the lipoma was not from within the rectus sheath or deeper. I did use a three-fourths-inch Penrose drain on that wound, and he healed perfectly! I had also had an older woman in the practice who had a large diastasis recti and abdominal redundant skin. On this lady, I did surgery as well and removed some abdominal skin. Although I was never completely happy cosmetically [because I had used interrupted stitches instead of continuous] with that surgery, she was thrilled. She too had no complications. I always calculated the toxic thresholds of injectable local anesthetics that we could use, and I did these procedures in my office. No need for hospital admission or exposure to megabugs.

When DV asked me to do an abdominal panniculectomy (tummy tuck) on her, she knew that I was capable. I asked if she had seen a plastic surgeon about it, and she said she had. She had been told of a huge and unmanageable fee. I have always felt so proud of my maternity patients, coping with life as their bodies get all stretched out. *I considered her request as therapeutic*: to encourage the next steps in her life, *not as frivolous*. The lawyer for the college characterized my willingness to help her as not maintaining appropriate boundaries with her. But I felt that way about ALL my "moms." If I could help them, I would want to do it. I know Counsel for the College would figure that meant not maintaining appropriate boundaries with all of my patients – by wanting the best for them. Even now, I think that we could design a procedure in a small site (approved by a college and its bylaws, of course) that would provide a good solution, of high quality, and appropriate safety without huge costs. But that's the way my mind thinks. I have a master's degree in experimental surgery. I did the procedure on her to enable her to go on to the best feelings about herself and move on in her life.

But I was not without fault:

- I did not place a surgical drain in the wound, relying instead on the pedicle of tissue coming up from the abdominal wall to the umbilicus as a "natural drain."
- My office had not been accredited for the procedure as a nonhospital surgical facility by the dumb new bylaw at that time. Now, although I have said that it was a dumb bylaw, this *was really too much* surgery for my small office setting. I should have declined to do the surgery in that setting.
- I did not attach a complete operative report to her chart but simply summarized things.
- I had to operate quickly because of the time constraints associated with a local anaesthetic, albeit with intravenous sedation. Having more time could well have contributed to a more bloodless field. I removed a curvilinear ellipse of tissue and brought her umbilicus (belly button) through a higher new site.

- I had only hand cautery and hand ties available for hemostasis (the control of bleeding), which also contributed to greater bleeding.

At that time I did surgeries in the office on Wednesdays, and that would give us two weekdays to watch for complications. She was OK when she came back in on Friday for a dressing change, but on Saturday, she had fainted and felt light-headed. She came out to the XXXX General Hospital where I was working emerg. I checked her blood haemoglobin, and it had dropped considerably. I arranged to transfuse two units of packed cells and, also, arbitrarily put her on an antibiotic. A few days later, a repeat blood test showed that her hemoglobin had come up nicely. We still had to deal with hematomas and seromas about like the care I had provided postoperatively following the breast-reduction surgeries.

Now, Danielle did fine in the end and is very happy with the cosmetic result of my work. Between you and me, I think the site looks SUPERB! She has gone on to become a surgical nurse, herself. It did work out! However, *I was in error* to expose her to such risk. Nonetheless, I strongly feel that *all women* who bring beautiful children to our world and country should have the option of this procedure being paid for. I suspect I won't earn a lot of brownie points among medical economists for that wish. Perhaps the children should eventually pay for their mom's surgery.

So having found this tidbit and pursuing it, the college suspended me for one month for this, as they had suspended my ex-senior partner for one month for having sex with his counseling patient. We were informed of, and anticipated the payment of, about $4,000 for costs to the college, but we were billed for more than $16,000. I had charged my patient $400 for my services. I can't say it paid well. But then, I was not like my ex-senior partner. I was never going to use medicine as my jumping-off point to profound wealth. Do you still keep in touch with RE, Mr. Registrar?

The investigating committee had made known its findings on the final four complainants on 10 February '05 and issued them on 7 April '05. I sought permission to change legal counsel, and it was finally granted. My new legal team (Dana and Deanna) requested a judicial review of the proceedings by the college because they believed that irreversible harm *had been done*. In December 2005, the Honorable Justice S. D. Hillier brought forward his findings. He said that many of our concerns were well-founded, but that he saw no issue that would keep the college from fixing its own mistakes. He felt that irreversible harm *had not yet occurred* and Counsel for the College wasn't about to emphasize to His Honor that the findings that the committee made could not be changed at that point. Nevertheless, we had found the *unfindable* witness, and so with a little hope we went back to the same panel as before. Not very surprisingly, they were a "hanging jury." This time they had to be very obtuse. They maintained the following:

- That I should have included in my "running commentary/ consent the phrase *"My left hand may make incidental contact with one or both of your breasts."* Do you suppose that anyone would say such a goofy thing?
- That *the found chaperone's evidence clarified nothing* as she could not remember if there was a manipulation done or not, or what *exactly the patient was wearing* those five years later. You'll remember from the transcript that she had, in fact, correctly remembered that a manipulation *WAS NOT DONE!* I can hardly believe that you folks chose to discredit Gaiana's memory because she couldn't recall WG's outfit four years later. Doesn't that embarrass you just a bit, as a feminist, Ms. Social Worker?
- That my providing the abdominal surgery to my ex-employee and maternity patient showed that I failed to maintain an appropriate doctor and patient boundary. As I have inferred, if being uncaring and unavailable is the appropriate patient boundary for *this college*, then I surely don't want to come under its dark shadow again.

- That they could not, in fact, modify their previous dumb findings loaded with sexual innuendo, grave concerns as to my motivations, and sinister intent.

I think they could have. *They could*, in fact, have said, *"We want to be an honorable committee and cannot, in good conscience, go on with this disciplinary hearing! We are simply unable to continue because of the now-obvious contradictions! We, with due respect, will have to return it to council!"* What stopped them? *Pride* and the need to be right.

- That "Dr Litchfield had been warned clearly by Dr Bear and Dr Flynne that *his method of examination of a female patient's back must include an explanation of the procedure and consent for skin to skin contact of sensitive female body areas as necessary components of his methodology* of examination," which, as you have read in chapter 2, was NOT their guidance! What was emphasized as you will note when you reread Dr. Bear's letter is that the only reference to skin-to-skin was with regard to having a chaperone.
- That PF's recall of the encounter must be much sharper than Gaiana Brooker's because the event happened in September and her complaint letter was created in January after her church friend made a complaint, and yet it wasn't until . . . well . . . January that Gaiana had been interviewed. So it must have been much more muddled in her mind because of the . . . huge . . . difference, . . . in elapsed time?! Okay. Well, the committee would like to ask that you not spend much time examining their logic here . . . as there really is none.
- That because they are proceeding to do violence against a physician, it is incumbent upon them to use *violent words* to describe his actions such as *nipple pinching*, instead of attempts to express *and bra removal*, instead of unclasping.
- That contrary to any printed literature on the subject, the piriformis muscle shall from now on be "easily [and separately] palpable from the buttock."

- Or, in the alternative, that the piriformis muscle can be palpated internally in a relaxed patient either via the vagina OR the rectum – without causing terrible harm.
- Page 12 of the committee's findings said that *my credibility suffered* "when he admitted he did not believe in promoting breast self examination in his patients, a widely accepted norm". *Not surprisingly they got this wrong too!* Page 515, lines 18 and on directly refute that finding with my testimony: that I do encourage and teach every woman to do it. Page 80 says that I did take the time to do it with PV – remember, first I do it and then I guide their hand so that they can do it . . . on one side, and then the other – pointing out that there should be mirror imagery of breast findings. And PV figured after one side of teaching, why would I do the other side? *You* actually remember, don't you?

The investigating committee may have been trying to find guilt in me by my reference on transcript page 639 where I refer to SBE (self breast exam) becoming a less certain medical recommendation from the academics. This information comes from Carolyn Pim, in *The Canadian Journal of CME*, July 2005, page 45 in the subsection "What About Breast Self-Examinations?" Dr. Pim was, then, the director of screening programs, Alberta Cancer Board, and a clinical assistant professor, Department of Community Health Sciences, the University of Calgary.

This fine panel suggested to council in the majority that I be suspended from practice for a year, and then allowed to do only surgical assisting; and in the minority, that I be erased from the registry. Council went with the "minority report."

Years ago, in the Midwest United States, small towns would get a pretty excited feeling that THEY KNEW some feller deserved to be hung. It happens, even to good people, when the Mob-ocracy feeling is afoot. Suddenly, each wants to contribute and "cast his stone." One of you is a family doctor, one is a pediatrician, and one is a social worker. These positions are respected in the community. Don't get caught up in lynching. It's exciting, but you really do know that it's wrong!

Council's order was in place as of the summer of 2007. We planned an appeal. We obtained an order suspending the order of the college on 12 September 2007 by the Honorable Mr. Justice Marceau, but he, in keeping with *possible* issues of protecting the public, restricted me from providing care to females age thirteen and older, pending the appeal. After he had learned that at any time since 2002's first complaint, the college had had the authority to suspend me from practice but had not felt it necessary; he actually commented that he felt like saying that I could just do everything just the way I had done before but figured that *the media would have a heyday with him*! Although my privileges in Edmonton hospitals were then limited to surgical assists at the Alex and the university hospitals, the *medical public* needed to have their say. The nurses at the university hospital surgical suite and one feisty little orthopedic surgeon refused to work with me, one day when I came in for my shift. After all, the college was now making known its findings – this brought a rising, general moral certitude about my nature as a predator. After all, the *college itself could never be wrong*! Not once! Not ever, right? So any offense any of them felt like dishing out must be deserved, right?

The limitation in my practice severely limited my income. We appealed. The appeal, though, does not allow a complete revisitation of all the facts and issues. It can only focus on legal error, real or suspected. It was hard to see enough patients to make ends meet. I felt I had let down my wife and family as provider. We lost the appeal, and immediately the order of council, now led by "appropriately promoted" *true-blue company man*, the chairman of my disciplinary committee – took effect at the close of my day on 6 May 2008. Erased from the register! As though I had never existed! Not for charges that I could grudgingly feel guilty about, but because of political moilings within the college – a chairman of investigation who became an assistant registrar, who became the registrar. He didn't apparently accept that attempted nipple expression was a part of a normal breast exam and got his indebted protégé to voice these personal views. It was irregular to use a specialist in that way, but something he figured he could get away with – except that their view was inconsistent with the World Medical view, notably the *New England Journal of Medicine*. All the rest was of lesser consequence, but if he could convince the committee that that one thing was an egregious affront to womankind, then he would have destroyed me . . . perhaps as a favor to . . . an old drinking buddy?

If such a person continues as registrar, it will be because the physicians of the province deserve him.

CHAPTER 8

WHAT WAS ESPECIALLY TORMENTING
AT THAT TIME?

B ETWEEN MY PREVIOUS trials in *criminal* court, the College of Physicians and Surgeons of Alberta decided that they needed to proceed with a disciplinary hearing in my regard. I had been in the newspapers. Hospital staff members talked about me. Radiology staff members talked about me, and one of them wanted to satisfy her personal desire for titillation by asking one of my pregnant patients, "Does Dr. Litchfield do a vaginal exam on you every time you go in?" I suppose she did not think of her own actions as harmful, but "just a healthy curiosity," or maybe her being "protective" of my patient. Her own lack of any real professionalism was just not an issue. My staff members were constantly assailed by their uninformed friends for even thinking of working in my office – for hadn't the media already established my guilt? I had already been convicted by public opinion, hadn't I? Court was only a formality!

As I have told you, we were informed that the Supreme Court of Canada had found in favor of the Crown – that we should have been required to present a defense. This was a blow to me and my family. Yet while the college had one request of me (to use a chaperone), *it continued to allow me* to practice medicine. I still had privileges at the Royal Alexandra Hospital and was doing deliveries there regularly. Dennis Kreptel, my department head (family practice) at the Alex interviewed me and alerted me that there were nurses on the station, who, although they had no real facts, thought that I should be "thrown to the lions." Remember what I said about medical people liking to be right? About forming opinions? If they told their parlor-room guests that I was certainly guilty, it must have been difficult to accept an actual court determining otherwise. 'Cause after all, "where there's smoke, there's fire!" Dr. Kreptel had told me that some of the nurses were gunning for me. They were my enemies. But of course, I did not ever know them by name. That let them "operate" in secret – and just spread their comments without ever having to be identified. Is this a part of the actual definition of pathetic? I have wondered whether the two nurses at the Alex, who were the last to complain about me (for rubbing a patient's thigh while she was in labor), had just remained "invisible" from that little group of "decided condemners" all the way from 1992? Rule of thirds, right?

Dr. Kreptel said that they felt I was "too familiar" with my patients. I asked him what that meant, and he told me that he didn't frankly know, either. I wondered if I was being told to be more distant from my patients, less available, less empathetic, less caring, just arriving at the last minute, or a bit too late – more like the "average doctor." Maybe they thought being caring and compassionate were a part of nurses' turf, and a doctor had no business meddling there. These, too, were hard thoughts because remember I'm a medical person too, and I like to be right, and do right by my view. I wondered if these *anonymous nurses* would eventually rise against me. I knew that with a one-person office, if ever, one of my own staff made a complaint against me, I would have no defense.

TRIBUTE TO MY STAFF

But my staff were noble and great supporters: Pam DeLuca, Karen Davidson, June Eeles, Kandice Layton (my sister-in-law), my wife Dianne, Rebecca Anderson (my daughter), Amy Jefferies (my daughter), Leisl Litchfield (my daughter), Kanoe Crowfoot, Nanna Hamilton, Barb Kreider, Julie Theunisse, and her sister Jennifer Theunisse! My youngest daughter Keltie also came with me at times, for calls into the office or a house call. And as long as I used a chaperone for exams at the office or the hospital, I would be safe in every other instance. Well, at least in theory, anyway! Oh, as long as I used a chaperone *AND* didn't allow inadequate gowning or covering. Just those two things, . . . oh, *AND* not removing bras, that's all – just those three things *AND* . . . (Remember Steve Martin in *The Jerk?*). No wait, in the final four, the college was saying that I hadn't exposed those patients *enough*! For the exams on them, I should have had the patients stark naked – so that my hand placement on them could clearly be seen by the chaperones. Do you get the feeling this was a no-win situation? Let all the chaperones see where your hands are by exposing your patients *more*?! But remember to adequately drape, so your patients are exposed *less*!

Because as the lawyer for the college says "what is even more telling, is that he did THIS while a chaperone was present," (page 152). THIS being – "his hand cupping the breast and the hand is hidden from the chaperone" (page 162). But wait, *that isn't the evidence* given by the actual witnesses, is it? That would be the "evidence" of the Counsel for the College? So did you lead your own evidence here? Did anyone get to cross-examine you? My lawyer and I must have missed that part of the hearing. Nevertheless, if you can object and sustain your own objections, then perhaps you can lead your own evidence and cross-examine yourself! But that isn't the evidence from any of the three witnesses: PV, PF, or WG! One of those witnesses describes assault before the nurse came in. The other two of those three witnesses said it was *both hands on their breasts at the same time* in front of the chaperone who must have missed the assault – one of these chaperones being my wife! Don't complain, counsel! It was you who ensured that they say that. Two hands, remember? And you tried to get my wife, too, to allow that you could be right. But now you're saying one unseen hand 'cause that kind of goes with the smoke you're trying to blow. Did you really think no one would ever go through these transcripts again? No chance anyone would catch *your* con? Or were you just tired of being a lawyer/judge? That third witness, according to the transcripts, said it was *one hand under the edge of the gown that she'd have been sitting on! And all this, before the chaperone entered the room* – unrelated to her exam! All three allegations of criminal assault but none describing one-handed breast cupping out of the direct sight of the onlooking chaperone. That was *only your evidence*, counsel! Did the committee accept your unwarranted conjecture? Really?

Think for a minute. Do you think that your breasts could be fondled from behind with someone's two hands at the same time, with another person in the room whose intent it was to observe, and that this could be missed? That is what the fine lawyer for the college wants you to believe. Be a CSI and block it out – choreograph it. Does it seem possible? Does it seem reasonable? Yeah . . . that's because it isn't reasonable!

HOW WAS I HURT?

We got the findings of the committee regarding their "judgement," if it can be called that, on the tenth of February 2005. My lawyer was fairly blunt with the results, but as I have said, he didn't consider me to be his client. Rather, my insurance company was his client. The thoughts that occurred to me were devastating. I still had schoolchildren. Our finances had been significantly compromised by WG's complaint that lost for me the supplemental income from rural emergency room shifts. I had assumed that since WG's complaint was so fallacious, a group of doctors like myself would easily see through it: I had had faith in them. I had been hoping for them, clear insight. I had been praying for them. I had such faith in my profession. These are educated people, I thought. I ought to feel comfortable in their hands. I had faced some harsh accusations in the past, and although it was very difficult, we had survived as a family. I trusted in the wisdom of the college because I felt I had chosen the best profession ever. I knew I had given up much of my own life and taken time from my family in order to serve medicine. I believed that my sacrifices were like those by others, and worth it in the end. I probably had unrealistic expectations about the nobility of the college. Here, I need to restate that the college is not the same as the Alberta or Canadian Medical Association. I found the AMA to be very supportive, and I accessed the AMA help line for both my wife and myself. It wasn't the AMA but the college that had let me down. I thought they were aware of all types of training in physical examination. They were, instead, just *not that knowledgeable*. I thought their memory of their previous judgment of my manual therapy assessment of the thoracic spine would still be on their file about me. They just *didn't clue in*! I had expected that expert witnesses – really all witnesses – would be honest, except for the WG complainant. She probably suffers a true inability to be honest with herself. I expected lies from her but was sure my fellow doctors would be able to see through them. I was disappointed in that too.

My blood pressure went up, and I began to have more of my familial "essential tremor" in my right hand. I began to stutter. That was a real blow because I had had some pride in my ability to speak. I still was doing full solo office practice with obstetrics, orthopedic surgical assisting, and extended care of my elderly. I could see that the findings of the committee were profoundly biased, wrong, and implied (again) sexual impropriety. That again meant that I was labelled unfaithful to my wife. That thought always made me sad. The previous assistant registrar, who had handled my case [the one who had defrauded the college] had asked me once WHY I should be so much complained of *if there wasn't strong foundation* for such complaints? What I told him, I still believe, it was because *I had been previously accused PUBLICLY!* It was out there IN THE COMMUNITY – like a bag of feathers emptied on a windy day, which can never be gathered back up! That was the reason. That was why I should be complained of further. When patients who didn't know me well were told of my past accusations; they naturally went over my encounters with them, with a fine-toothed comb, asking themselves: had they ever felt uncomfortable or embarrassed? Well, yes. The practice of medicine deals with very personal things, and that includes sexuality. Some probably felt that I should announce to each of them my past accusations, though unproven, when they first met me. How foolish that would have been. Perhaps the committee – well, especially the social worker – even felt that I should say right off. "My name is Dr Litchfield. In the past, I have been accused of fondling my patients' breasts and vaginas, of overly exposing them in exams, and kissing them soundlessly in the midst of exams. *Welcome to my practice.*" What a kooky, awkward way to start a professional relationship. I knew that those accusations had been false. I had suffered through seven years of criminal court over them. I wanted to forget them.

I knew that some nurses at my hospital still carried grudges after I had been judged not guilty. I didn't know which ones those nurses were, but I did notice a lack of cooperation occasionally. They probably felt that *any patient who believed in me* didn't deserve their "best care": their A game! [That really has less to do with me than it has to do with them, doesn't it?] Some fairly frequently tried to "create" a situation in which transfer of care to a specialist seemed appropriate. Some called me late for deliveries. But they would never declare themselves openly. They worked behind the scenes, in the *secret tradition* of the greatest gossips. I often had to go to the hospital as soon as the patient got there in order to confirm that the information that was being transferred to me was correct. On occasion, they would call me in "too late" for a delivery, initiating the call after the delivery had occurred. At least once while I was in the family doctor's on-call room sleeping, they failed to call me when my patient had difficulties – even though I was just down the hall – and they simply made a referral to a specialist! The nurse at the desk defiantly asked, "Well, what would you have done?" My answer was, "I'd have called the attending physician – me!"

They probably felt some sense of being justified in compromising the physician/patient relationship that my patients had with me because they knew *the real gossip, I mean, their real truth*! Somehow, that was justifiable to them. One of them made a complaint to the college that in the course if a labor and delivery, I had rubbed the thigh of a patient in discomfort whose knees were not staying apart while she was bearing down. The patient and her family were lifelong friends of mine. The patient had no complaint, just the nurse. It was very fleeting, apparently, although I have no clear idea of what I was actually being accused of, or when this may have occurred. She had been charting and glanced over and saw me apparently rubbing the inner right knee or thigh of this patient. When the college had gone out to the hospitals to recruit complaints about me, they had come up with this gem. What a find! The patient's husband and family had not complained, and they disagreed with the accusation of inappropriateness in my care to their daughter/wife. The patient did as well. But there was a disciplinary hearing for this obscure complaint as well. The three members of this committee, however, led by Blaire Paxton (a lawyer) *found me not guilty* of unbecoming conduct. The decision of that honest disciplinary committee was not good enough, however, for the registrar and his cronies. They got the Council of the College to reverse the findings of that committee and declare me guilty based on their heap of already accumulated findings with regard to the four complainants who actually did complain in this final barrage.

After the judicial review, that hearing committee heard evidence from the additional witnesses, including the "lost and found" nurse, Gaiana Brooker. *Right after* hearing Gaiana's evidence – *immediately after* – the artful college counsel *made clear* to the committee that they did not have the right to change their original findings. Why was that? Why so immediate? Because she had been convincing! He knew their conclusions were incorrect and perhaps that the committee was then having misgivings. I'll bet he laughed at the thought of sticking it to Judge Hillier – he had finessed the judge who had said that the college could get it right! So the disciplinary committee proceeded in September 2006 to evidence and submissions on penalty with the belief that they had *no jurisdiction to consider* new evidence with regards to the findings that they had erroneously already made. Remember they still wanted to be right because . . . well, you know the routine! Golly, *they would be embarrassed if their damning findings were linked to a lenient penalty*! From September 2006 to spring 2007 they considered. Then I was called on the telephone by my lawyer one day in the spring of 2007 and told that I had to stop practicing that night. But we would, of course, appeal.

We were back in court in September 2007 to seek my renewed practice, pending appeal. I briefly regained the temporary privilege to practice medicine except on females over age twelve, pending the results of an appeal. Appeals are not what lay people think they are. They do not allow a complete revisiting of the entire case – they only allow a legal examination of errors in law. They don't permit discussion of the things that I have shown you were unethical from the start. No judge or group ever knew that expert 1 had *clearly taken sides, excluded evidence, and gave an alternative to her previous statement under oath* as an expert witness; nor that expert 2 had allowed that his criteria for inappropriateness were actually just based on *differences from his clinical method.* If it was unnecessary for his method (with patient lying on tummy), *he allowed legal counsel* to paint the difference as *inappropriate* for me, with the patient upright. He did not do upright exams of the thoracic spine and therefore did not see how essential counterpressure against the sternum was, in doing it this way. He did not do pelvic exams in assessment if he thought them necessary, but instead referred them out – so they *must* be wrong too?!

From September to December 2007, in addition to taking antidepressants from my family doctor, I started to see a psychologist – paid for by the AMA. Around Christmas of 2007, the AMA's physicians-in-crisis team came to my home. A psychiatrist did a house call to me from Calgary! She then arranged to have me seen by a very kind local psychiatrist. I continued the sleep meds and antidepressants that my family doctor had started me on.

The "appeal" came and we lost. Again, the day I got the news, I had to stop practicing. So I closed my practice on May 6, 2008. But I continued to go in there every day to clean things up, shred sufficiently old charts, throw away my beloved textbooks of medicine, and be present *for those of my patients who wished to pick up their charts and weep with me.* Some of them just needed to hug me and say good-bye. Every day, more patients would come and grieve with me. The grief would restart fresh with each day. Mostly, we knew we were saying farewell, forever. Like the first baby I had delivered in Edmonton, who still enjoyed getting stickers for being good, when she came in for her own prenatal visits. Every patient had a story that I remembered. Seeing twenty-four to thirty-five patients per day for twenty years in my solo practice meant that I had been seeing a lot of fine people with whom I had formed relationships. Many wanted me to find for them a physician like me. I wasn't sure I would be able. When Dianne and I had moved to Barrie, Ontario, we went to the hospital's chief of obstetrics to talk about finding a family doctor. He only asked one question, Do you want your family doctor to be very involved with your family, or just do medicine and leave the rest alone. He talked of Calgary and McMaster being different than the rest. We chose involvement, and he referred us to Dr. Brian Morris. Brian was the best family doctor we had ever known. He was great with the kids and knowledgeable/conscientious. I wanted to be like Brian, but I am sure he would easily be accused of being too familiar with his patients. If I can't be involved like that, I'd just as soon not do medicine. I think that being involved is what made me a committed doctor and want to keep current, do CME, and acquire more skills. I thought that's what medicine was. And I really think that I am not the only doctor like me. Hopefully, a further college witch hunt will not burn them out of our community.

I had to let my staff go. I had no way to commemorate my gratitude to them for their loyalty and support. I had to throw away most of my medical textbooks – so much appreciated as a forum for learning. There was no place for them at home, especially as it appeared that I would never need them again, and we were going to be bankrupted and lose our home from the costs of the proceedings against me – $170,000 the fee for their service of emotional rape, career destruction, and endangering the lives of my wife and myself. I still had a few loonies in my change purse, but it was not close to enough. I had to throw away some furniture and equipment, sell some at garage sale prices, and take just a bit home. I could not rent a place to store charts because I had no income. Still there was overhead.

We were going to lose our home. I was told I had to pay for the office until the end of July. I wanted to be out of the office by the end of June. I was busy shredding old charts, giving away what little I had left. I was seeing my psychiatrist and taking an antidepressant. Also, I was taking the same medications at night that my family doctor had prescribed for sleep. I was taking medication for my blood pressure. I had needed nighttime sedatives in order to have any sleep for about a year up to that point. Still some nights I did not sleep at all anyway. I just lay there, motionless. I thought of the many, many times Dianne and the children had forfeited time with me so that I could serve MEDICINE. She was a tough mistress – medicine. And now, this – the sting of the college labelling of implied sexual impropriety. From the same group who had slapped the wrist of my former senior partner for a clearly more egregious sexual encounter. But I got up in the mornings and went in to the office. I tried not to waken Dianne when I left because of the apparent peace that came to her in sleep. She was my truest and most loyal friend. I am so unsure that I will ever have a partner again.

I was socially withdrawn. I would go to church but hope that no one asked me to speak, sing, teach, or pray. I was becoming hollow. My dear wife carried me metaphorically, though her own health was not good. She was on a beta-blocker to slow down her heart rate. She took medicine for depression and asthma. She was saddened at my loss of desire for intimacy because it really did allow us to *"be as one."* She would encourage me to have faith. She would encourage me to eat. She would encourage me to go on. She would encourage me to be freer with my shopping. She *WAS* my encouragement. She still wanted to share with me. At that point, she wanted to share with me excerpts from *So You Think You Can Dance*, ice skating, or *Dancing with the Stars*, but we didn't go to movies anymore (our past solace – could you tell from my references?) due to the cost and my anxiety being out, in public. Dianne provided simple meals and continued to run the house and the finances. She had one knee replacement early in 2007 and the second one in March 2008.

Before the first general anaesthetic, her internal medicine doctor wanted her heart fully checked out. She saw cardiology and eventually even had a cardiac catheterization and coronary angiogram. That checks for narrowing in the coronary arteries. Her coronaries were flawless, so she went ahead with the anaesthesia and surgeries. One son served a mission and returned. A daughter left to serve as a missionary in Uruguay. I had difficulty spending any money because I worried for our future. I would skimp on groceries and only buy the least expensive things. I would eat very little. I was no fun. *I so wish I had bought more flowers for Dianne.* I didn't enjoy life. I thought of death frequently. I hoped that by dying, somehow my family would be provided for. I felt that I was a burden. I lost considerable weight starting at 242 lbs and ending at 170 lbs. My muscle mass was reduced to virtually nothing. I was unsteady on my feet, and I fell down at times. I certainly had no appetite. I *didn't want to hear my last name or my title* out loud in public because I had failed in continuing to be able to provide for my dear family, and *having the title of doctor didn't seem to have much honor, anymore.* I didn't want to be recognized by anyone but my family. I wore baggy, faded, unnoticeable clothes. I avoided any noisy places and shopped when stores were least busy. It was even taxing to have my precious grandchildren over. I was becoming used up. I understood hell. It wasn't *being unable* to be with those you love; it was *Not wanting* to be with those you love.

On the night of June 26, 2008, four days before the office was to be empty, I took medication to try to sleep in anticipation of an appointment the next day. I held motionless in bed for very long periods. I could not sleep, so I took more medicine, then more. I was definitely drugged and not thinking clearly, but not sleeping. In my blur, I took all the medication I had – an "intentional overdose." I don't recall right then having wanted to die, but I did want to sleep for a long time, to escape the pain and the unfairness. Perhaps twelve hours later, my wife and eighteen-year-old son attempted to waken me with shaking and ice water; I can sort of recall being aware of that. I was taken to the Grey Nuns Hospital by an ambulance. I was in and out of consciousness for days. Things were very blurry. Me – in emergency – where I had spent so much time working. I had acquired an aspiration-type pneumonia somehow. My dear wife and a few friends came to visit me. That is pretty blurry.

I found myself in psychiatric unit 91 a while later. Each day, I was to wake up, shave, shower, and dress by nine for the breakfast cart's arrival. That was the routine. Some mornings, I sluggishly did *part* of the routine. Other mornings I slept in, and the nurses occasionally came to feed me because *my hands shook* so much – I spilled a lot. Very slowly and gradually I adopted the hospital routine. God bless the Grey Nuns Hospital Department of Psychiatry. They helped me so much! Dr. Mills, my in-hospital psychiatrist, did not start me in group therapies with the other patients initially. I don't know if he thought the *other patients* would *fear* me because of rekindled publicity, or if he thought that he would try not to *embarrass me* by requiring my participation in group therapies. I was Dr. Litchfield. That was my name, but I didn't want it. I had overdosed. I could not support my family. In this assault, I brought shame to my family name. I had gotten as low as I could get – I had hit bottom. They allowed me out on overnight and weekend passes with Dianne, but sometimes I was too anxious to stay in my own home, and I had to come back to the "safety" of the hospital early. Although she was still recovering from her second total knee replacement and was not very mobile, Dianne came and visited me regularly at the hospital, or came to bring me home for passes. I was five weeks as inpatient. About the third week, I began to realize that I needed to start to talk with others. I convinced Dr. Mills that I really had to do group therapies like everyone else, even though it frightened me. At the end of this admission, my last name would still be *Litchfield*. And I would still be a doctor, although no longer licensed. Those were things I could not really change.

But I started to want to live.

I began to want to get better. I was taking a ton of medicine. I started to go to *exercise group*. I began to rebuild some muscle. Exercise helped me establish routines. Routine is so important at that point in depression – whether it comes from within or without. I ventured with exercise and craft group OUTSIDE the protection of the hospital walls. I was taken off constant suicide watch. They let me have my belt back and shoelaces. I began to talk more. I participated in groups. The staff had to caution me because I was rediscovering social appropriateness. I really didn't know how to act. We wondered if I was going "hypomanic." That subsided but did not evaporate. They eventually released me from inpatient to the outpatient psychiatric program; that meant that I came to the hospital from 9:00 to 16:00 hrs. From this too, I was formally released on 17 September 2008. Dianne was at my side.

I began to try to *be of help to her.* My depression and anxiety was coming under control with the medication. I was in my home. I was with my family. We declared bankruptcy on 21 October 2008. We could not possibly pay our bills in closing the office and the $170,000 that the college demanded as costs for its *unjust proceedings against me.* Cameron came home from his mission in Toronto at the beginning of November. Leisl was a missionary in Uruguay, and Marcus left as a missionary to Argentina. Each had earned the money required to support themselves as missionaries, except for the occasional small need that they still looked to their father for. With Dianne's blessing, I started to do online training in clinical research and started looking for some kind of job. I needed one that didn't require handwriting or any other task that required a steady right hand. If I was late with my medication, I would get jittery and stutter. I began to trust myself to drive again. It is very hard to get any job. Any check on my previous employment made me not that desirable as an employee. Marcus did leave as a missionary for Argentina. I had David, Cameron, and Keltie at home with Dianne and me. I asked that my disability insurance provide the agreed support, but it was not until January of 2009 that this began, albeit retroactively. At some point I anticipated that there would be an issue about me being unable to function in my own occupation – because my licence had been removed, after all. Keltie was in grade 11 and was not hitting it off well with her stressed mother. I was pretty useless as a parent. David and Cameron were really quite independent and had found close, dear girlfriends, whom they each eventually married.

On the evening of Sunday, November 23, 2008, I was on the computer doing more of my online training so that I could find some employment. *Dianne was sprawled on our bed* across the hall chatting with me. Then she decided to call her parents and just chat with them. They were so dear. I loved the sound of her voice when she was on the phone with them. She was peaceful. Dianne and I had started kissing again, just for practice. It was fun! She was the very BEST! I woke up that night at three thirty or so. We slept beside each other, and because of her acid reflux, we had a wedge right across the whole upper portion of the bed to raise our heads. Some nights as she slept, she would turn so that her body would be in a mound at the bottom of the wedge. That would make her breathing more rough, so I would help her reposition herself to lying properly on our wedge. I did that, that night at 3:30 a.m. I went to the washroom and came back to lie beside her and sleep again. With the medication I was on, I could *sleep every night* and have some energy in the day. [It was Seroquel, among many others.] With Dianne's help, I could feel myself healing. My nonhospital psychiatrist and family doctor were so helpful too. I enjoyed my Scripture reading and prayers again.

I woke up just after 05:00 hrs on Monday the twenty-fourth of November. I didn't know why I woke up. Then I realized, I couldn't hear Dianne breathing. I quickly reached over to her and was relieved to find her warm and soft, like usual. Then I realized that she was not breathing. And I could not hear heart sounds with my ear to her chest! Our room was totally dark because we have shutters on the window.

In that total dark, I quickly became *Dr. Litchfield* again. I began CPR. I did the best CPR there has ever been on this earth! My compulsive technique was flawless. While doing chest compressions, I would call out to her and encourage her to awaken. I prayed loudly. My noise woke up my sixteen-year-old daughter across the hall. She came in and turned on my light. Dianne's dear lips were blue. "OH NOOO! That's not good," my inner self said. But I kept doing CPR. I moved my lips against hers to breathe for her. She was still warm, maybe there was a chance. I asked that Keltie call 911 for an ambulance and that she wake up the brothers in the basement. They came up and together provided a priesthood blessing to Dianne while I kept doing CPR. My kids could have participated in the CPR because they have learned a few things in my home, but I wanted to do it myself. So that I knew that it was done perfectly. I still had my OCD.

Surprisingly soon we were joined by fire truck and ambulance crews. I reluctantly allowed them to replace me. For a time they did this in my bed – starting IVs and putting on the electrodes for the heart monitor. The doctor part of me listened to the monitor electronic voice inform us that hers was not an appropriate situation for defibrillation because she had NO heart rhythm. The team took her to the firmer surface of my dining room laminate floor, where I knelt at her side. My son Shawn and his wife, MariClaire, came over. Shawn knelt across from me and began singing the primary songs that Dianne had taught the children. I joined him in singing, as best I could. The crew leader informed me that the medications had not helped, and that at no time had she had any heart rhythm (electrical activity). They said that we should stop. They said that my fifty-three-year-old wife of thirty-two years, Dianne, was dead. I think my own heart stopped too. *I'm not sure it has ever restarted.* But it still aches, so maybe that pain is "proof of life."

I go on each day and, from Tom Hanks's *Sleepless in Seattle,* "*remind myself to breathe*" and eat and shower and shave and exercise and dress. I am reminded of the first exchange between William Thatcher and the naked Geoffrey Chaucer in the movie *A Knight's Tale* (seeing a naked man on the road), "Oi sir, what are you doing?" Chaucer: "Uh … trudging. You know, trudging? [*Pause*] *To trudge: the slow, weary, depressing yet determined walk of a man who has nothing left in life except the impulse to simple soldier on.*" (From: *A Knight's Tale* – Wikiquote.)

I had to participate in Dianne's funeral and burial. I could not afford a tombstone for her grave because I had been bankrupted by the college's insistence that we pay for their violation of us and by my lesser bills in closing the office. She had no tombstone, but I had one made and put in place as of May 2010.

I had to figure out how to live and provide for David, Cameron, and Keltie who were still at home, plus Leisl and Marcus who were honorably serving missions in Uruguay and Argentina, respectively. We were entering the Christmas month. I was reeling. I had to figure out what the finances were like. Dianne had always done them and prepared tax stuff for our accountant. I wanted to give some kind of token gift to Dianne at Christmas, so I finished my course and wrote the online exam for my Clinical Research Associate Diploma on Christmas Eve 2008 at 18:25 hrs (I'm still a little bit military). I had given her the gift of my commitment to trudge on and somehow find a way to provide for my family.

Evan Esar said, "Character is what you have left when you've lost everything you can lose." Martin Luther King, in his gentle voice of peaceful opposition, said, "The ultimate measure of a man is not where he stands in moments of comfort and conscience, but where he stands at times of challenge and controversy." Dianne and I had been secretly pleased that the College of Some Physicians and Two Surgeons would not be getting their $170,000 blood money from us. We just didn't have that kind of money. As I became fully aware of the finances, I found an automatic withdrawal each month that I didn't know anything about. I discovered that in 1991, Dianne had got a life insurance policy for herself listing me as the beneficiary. With the check that eventually came, I became able to pay all my debtors. My bankruptcy was dissolved into a proposal 1, with the stipulation that all my debtors would be paid in full. They have been, including the $170,000 to the college – so that they can continue to provide "ethical guidance to the profession." What irony!

I don't have much left, but I have a home for my family, and I am able to provide a little for them. And now my head has cleared. I exercise every morning except the Sabbath, and I do yoga once or twice a week under the eye of my wife's aunt Judy, who is wonderful! I am starting to do little things, like distributing all-natural, high-impact health products to people through an online business, prune trees, and work in a bakery.

I can think clearly again. I can figure things out. My lawyer had me go through the steps of producing the undertakings which we had accepted in the Civil Litigation Process Examination for Discovery. I had to look things up. When I went through the college transcript from which I have quoted liberally, I found that *their entire process was flawed*. How that saddened me!

Now, Mr. Registrar, new assistant registrar, college investigator, hearing committee, and Counsel for the College, I have managed to get across your swamp! I have actually survived the holocaust of your trial of me. Your accusatory process has publicly raped me, but I am alive! My name is Bryant Litchfield, and *I am a Doctor!* Maybe the public didn't know *before* how you folks, individually or as a gang, define *"ethical guidance" to the profession*. I think your pictures need to be in the newspapers. I think your images need to be on television. There is corruption at work here. Not down in some vague South American country, but right here in Canada! Where will the "media" be on this one? Well, of course, it will always be where the story is. That, at least will never change. They may want to talk to the players in this production. Only this time I am not fettered in sharing my side of the issues and their ethics, and I think this story is evolving more into one about the registrar and the college traditions that may well be traditional but are not necessarily ethical.

So the antagonists and the protagonist stand. I have a disabling tremor so that I can't practice medicine as I was doing, ever again, but *"I'm not dead yet!"* as they say in Monte Python's *In Search of the Holy Grail*. Surely there is not a single one of you who feels justified in this proceeding against me. It certainly has harmed me, my wife, my family, my patients, and the community at large. When I took too much medication, I could well have died. My wife's heart did break and stop. Those of you involved who are medical, is this not what we took an oath about: ABOVE ALL, TO DO NO HARM? Whatever does our OATH mean to you?

CHAPTER 9

WHY I FELT SINGLED OUT AND BULLIED

I DID GRADES 1, 2, and 3 in two years. That meant that I was small for my grade. In grade 4, I began with excellent grades. My family was not wealthy, so we pretty well relied on our imaginations for entertainment. I took to taking apart ballpoint pens and using that clicker thing on the end as a rocket ship that could separate in stages. I then reassembled the pen and used it, but even when the clicker thing was covered in a chromed cap, there was a plastic bipartite or tripartite mechanism under the cap – and those plastic pieces were of different colors! It was so much fun to get a new pen and take it apart to see the different colors! However, as I said my family was not wealthy, so I picked up discarded or dropped pens wherever I walked. I would have wanted to be terribly honest and find every single owner of those pens, but I discovered that there is just no way to find pen owners. If I didn't pick them up, I would generally notice them a few days later scrunched by some car tire, including the "spaceship" in the clicker. I learned to be very assiduous in looking for and preserving the special spaceships. Most I kept with me in a narrow pickle jar that I kept in my metal school lunch box. Grade 4 at Allan Watson Elementary School in Lethbridge, Alberta, and the owner of a fleet of spaceships! Wow, was I lucky! Occasionally I would show my collection to a young friend. I was proud of my fleet.

Well, as it turns out, a girl in my class reported her ballpoint pen *stolen*, although she had probably dropped it. I didn't have any clue about that 'cause I had never stolen anything! The teacher said we couldn't go home 'til it was returned, and she had the principal come in. Woe, the principal – the pressure on the class increased. Finally, a fellow in the class to whom I had showed my collection said that he had seen the girl's pen in a bottle in my lunch box. I was briskly required to show my lunch box, and the pen was actually there. I was as surprised as anyone. Quicker than a flash, I was required to accompany the principal down to his office where I was lectured, reprimanded, and then given the strap sixteen times on each hand – eight for lying to everyone and eight for stealing. My violin hands! This was done by someone in authority. I knew he was wrong, but I just couldn't figure out how he could be and still be the principal of the school. That year I got the first D grade anyone in my family had ever had. It was the only one I ever got too because the next year, in grade 5, Ms. Neville was my teacher, and she liked music, and that was something my family and I did lots of. She was my favorite teacher; maybe because I felt accepted by her, and maybe because I had a small crush on her.

Now what does that vignette have to do with my current account? The registrar was a person in authority who had proclaimed that I was "proven guilty" of those charges cited at the beginning of the next chapter. I knew he was wrong, but I just couldn't figure out how he could be, and still be, the registrar of the college. So I did a little research of my own.

There are actually at least 411 published textbooks of physical exam. College expert 1 wrote AT THE START of this debacle: "Older methods of clinical breast examination do suggest that the nipples be checked for discharge, but this practice has been largely abandoned, as it serves no useful purpose." [I still have a copy of that letter.] She then went on to say "under oath" that that was not true and that she had only been giving me *the benefit of the doubt.* So which is it, Mme L'Expert? And is it possible that as an expert that you have only informed yourself of *one of the 411* approaches to physical examination? Would *YOU* consider that an admirable literature search? It is true that the Barbara Bates' *Guide to Physical Examination and History Taking,* tenth edition, by Lynn S. Bickley – published in 2009 by Lippincott, Williams, & Wilkins – refers to doing nipple expression only when a complaint of SPONTANEOUS nipple discharge has been reported. But wait, there are other methods! Do you think that the Bates text is the ONLY source; hence, the one that all physicians everywhere should be obliged to adhere to? When I originally spoke with the assistant registrar, I made him completely aware of the sources of my technique. Either he just couldn't explain them very well to the chairman of the complaints department (now registrar), or one or both of them decided that legitimate medical sources were unimportant to what they wanted to do.

Well, now, registrar and expert 1, I have something to say to you together. Here it is, quoting just myself, I guess "*transient, recent methods of clinical breast examination do suggest that the nipples need not be checked for expressible secretions, unless there is a some complaint of spontaneous discharge, but this trend in practice is being largely abandoned, as it serves to neglect potential pathology.*"

When the two of you brought your production to the stage of my disciplinary hearing, you really made me doubt myself. I knew from whence my training had come, but, Ms. Expert, you talked with such bravado that you made me doubt its validity. I doubted myself because you told your lie so effectively. The 1976 DeGowin and DeGowin text was, in 2004, called DeGowin's Diagnostic Examination, eighth edition. It was edited by Richard F. LeBlond, Richard L. DeGowin, and Donald D. Brown and published by McGraw-Hill. *The portion on breast exam had not changed!* Remember my disciplinary hearing happened in 2005, so the 2004 edition would have been pretty darned current. Professor DeGowin was, in 2005, an emeritus professor and no longer actively practicing. So after the hearing turmoil in 2007,

I called doctors Richard LeBlond and Donald Brown each on the phone. It took me a few days to get through to them. When I spoke with Dr. Brown, he said that he and his team were starting work on the next edition of the book. He was sensitive to the claims that spontaneous discharge was a more glaring clinical sign of cancer; he thanked me for raising the issue with him and his team and said they would consider making a change. Then I spoke with Dr. Richard LeBlond. He was such a gentleman and highly knowledgeable too! I frankly asked him if, for all these years, I had been mistaken about the direction that this fine textbook seemed to give. *He told me on the phone that I had gotten it right!* He said he would send me a letter on the subject. When I got his written response, it could not be used in an appeal because appeals don't go back to basic evidence, only how the law was applied. Here is Dr. LeBlond's letter to me:

> University of Iowa
> Health Care
>
> February 1, 2007
>
> Bryant Litchfield, MD
> #203, 8708 – 165 Street [The office that I closed in May, 2008]
> Edmonton, Canada, T5R 1W2
>
> Dear Dr Litchfield:
>
> I apologize for being so slow getting this letter out to you. Our conversation stimulated a lot of thought, once again, on the purposes and appropriate training and practice of physical examination. I am going to take a fairly longwinded stab at addressing the particular issue that you raised regarding breast examination.
>
> As with all observations, the interpretation of the observation depends upon the context. The context for our physical exam observations come from the history. It is the patient's

history, including family and social history, as well as past medical history, that allow us to create a hypothesis and also assign each hypothesis a clinical probability prior to the physical examination. The physical exam is a structured method of observation in which the anatomy and physiology of the body are observed by inspection, auscultation, percussion and palpation. The purpose of any particular physical examination is specific to the clinical context. This is important to keep in mind for the purposes of our discussion. The screening physical examination is quite different from the organ or system specific examination in a patient with complaints or signs specific to that system.

The physical exam is a structured sequential series of observations. It is important, and often misunderstood, that the *most difficult determination on the physical exam is normal.* The range of normal far exceeds the range of abnormal for most findings and flagrantly abnormal findings are easy for even the most inexperienced of examiners to detect. It is the observations at the margin between the broad range of normal and the near edge of abnormal that requires experience and expertise for interpretation. To this end, the more experience that *every examiner* has at exploring these margins, the more able they will be able to accurately make the difficult clinical judgements about what signs and symptoms require further evaluation, and which do not.

Now, as to the specific question of the appropriateness of the various parts of the breast examination: the breast exam, like all parts of the physical examination, is a skill acquired by performing a complete and full examination on *each and every* patient at the appropriate time intervals. Examination of the breasts requires inspection during various manoeuvres as well as palpation. *Part of breast palpation is palpation of the nipple and areola and gentle compression of the breast and nipple checking for galactorrhea.* [These are expressible secretions.

I think you'll recognize my technique here.] Galactorrhea and nipple discharges are not abnormal and by themselves may be of no particular significance. However, this can only be determined on the basis of the clinical history and *comparison with the other breast.* Certainly, all physicians and medical students in training, and physicians early in their career *should be adept* at each of these manoeuvres. It is, therefore, important that students be taught to do this and then be taught the sequential judgements required for correct interpretation. If this is not done, then, when confronted with a breast discharge or galactorrhea, *they will have no base of comparison* with which to compare their findings or the complaints of their patient. In the routine screening exam, I think this is *an appropriate manoeuvre* that adds insignificant time and no significant patient discomfort if the patient is properly instructed on the purpose of the examination. Breast examination should always be done with a female chaperone.

Extrapolation of this argument could lead one to think that the only reasonable screening examination is a head to toe reprise of all of the complete full systems examinations. This is not the case. There is not time to do all that. On the other hand, simple exams, such as examining the nipples appropriately, proper examination of neck veins, proper palpation of the precordial impulse, and examination of the male nipples, to name just a few, are parts of the routine screening examination that can be performed in seconds and add depth and useful information to the physical examination.

I apologize for the longwinded answer, but there is an old saying that for every complex question, there is a simple solution, and it is wrong. This is a complex and difficult question that requires a sophisticated understanding of the diagnostic process, the purpose of taking a complete history and physical examination, and the experiential base necessary for physicians to make appropriate clinical judgements. The most counter intuitive part of this is the difficulty of judging what is normal on a physical examination. I teach my students and residents that there are many, many normal people but no normal physical examinations. I have yet to see an individual who does not have an abnormality of some sort on physical examination, trivial though it may be. The difficulty is always, particularly as people age and develop more issues, the distinction between what is trivial and what is significant. This can only be done through experience, multiple sequential observations of a standardized history and physical exam over many years.

Thank you for raising this issue. I hope you find this essay useful.

Sincerely,

Richard F. LeBlond, MD
Professor, Clinical Internal Medicine

Can you not feel his gentle nature through these written words? This man is a good man. He is willing to take time from a busy schedule to reach out to a struggling family doctor: first on the phone and then in writing. He also invited me to come and visit him in Iowa. His text touches on the facts that

1. disease cannot be fully understood by access to just those without the disease, and
2. disease cannot be fully understood by access to just those with the disease.

But remember I said I had also had a conversation with Donald D. Brown, another of the editors. He'd said they would reassess that particular portion of the book and make decisions about it. So now, this is me quoting from their *DeGowin's Diagnostic Examination*, ninth edition, published in 2009 by McGraw-Hill:

> Nipple Examination
> Inspect the anterior trunk for supernumerary nipples. Look for fissures, scaling, excoriation, retraction or deformity of the nipple; recent deformities suggest acquired disease. Nipple discharge may be detected by gently compressing the nipple and areola between the thumb and the forefinger; this has not [yet] *proven* to be productive for cancer screening. Palpate the periphery of the areola for tenderness, nodules, or cords.
> The total time to complete a thorough breast examination should be approximately 6 to 10 minutes. An additional portion of the examination should include palpation of the axillary and supraclavicular fossae, searching for lymphadenopathy.

You will notice the part about nipple discharge having been modified *but still* being recommended. *Iowa still believes!* Is Iowa alone – the only place on the whole earth to recommend practice this way? Is Iowa sinister, dubious, and suspect as I have been described to be?

Well, let me quote to you from *Clinical Examination*, sixth edition, by NJ Talley and S O'Connor published by Elsevier in 2010. This comes *from Australia*. Under the portion on the breasts, page 436:

PALPATION

> Examine both the supraclavicular and axillary regions for lymphadenopathy. It may be difficult, however, to distinguish an axillary fat pad from an enlarged lymph node.
> Then ask the patient to lie down. The examination can be performed only if the breast tissue is flattened against the

chest wall. If the breasts are large, it can be helpful to have the patient place her hand on her forehead for the palpation of the lateral aspect of the breast and bring her elbow up level with the shoulder for the palpation of the medial side of the breast.

Palpation is performed gently with the pulps of the middle three fingers parallel to the contour of the breast. Feel the four quadrants of each breast systematically (Figure 14.2a). Don't pinch the breast as you may think you then feel a mass. The total examination should involve a rectangular area bordered by the clavicle, sternum, mid-axillary line and the bra line. Start in the axilla and palpate in a line down to the bra line inferiorly. The pattern of palpation is like that of mowing a lawn, a series of vertical strips that cover the whole of the rectangle (Figure 14.2b).

Each area is palpated three times, using small circular movements and slightly increasing pressure. Palpation is more difficult when a breast implant is present. It is probably best to examine such a patient in a supine position and to keep the ipsilateral arm down at her side.

Next feel behind the nipple for lumps and *note if any fluid can be expressed*: bright blood (from a duct papilloma, fibroadenosis or carcinoma), yellow serous (fibroadenosis), or serous (early pregnancy) fluid, milky (lactation) or green (mammary duct ectasia) fluid.

Don't mistake normal breast structures for a mass. You may feel a rib or costochondral junction normally on deep palpation. The inferior ridge of breast tissue (inframammary fold) may be felt and is symmetrical. You may feel normal rubbery-type plaques (fibroglandular tissue), especially in the upper outer quadrant. It is normal to feel firm breast tissue at the areola border."

So *in Australia*, nipple expression is being taught as a part of a regular complete breast exam! Is the whole island/continent guilty of unbecoming conduct? Next come with me to Tucson, *Arizona*, and a text by Jane Orient: *Sapira's Art and Science of Bedside Diagnosis*, the fourth edition, published by Lippincott, Williams, and Wilkins [You can always tell that a book has had some success when it gets along in its number of editions] – also in 2010:

Discharge from the Breast

A discharge from the nipples is very common in premenopausal women. In an ambulatory population, it was found in 13% of nulligravida and 22% of parous women between the ages of 16 and 50. Prolonged lactation was the most common cause (29% of cases). No definite cause was found in 43% of 586 cases (Newman et al, 1983). Nipple discharge alone is a RARE presenting symptom for carcinoma, occurring in less than 3% of patients (Chaudary et al, 1982). Coversely, of patients with a nipple discharge, 5.9% (Chaudary et al, 1982) to 13.3% (Leis et al, 1988) were found to have carcinoma.

Serous or Bloody Discharge

A serous or bloody discharge from the nipple can result from a wide variety of causes (Atkins and Wolf 1964; Barnes, 1966). Benign causes include fibrocystic disease, duct papilloma, papillary cystadenoma, chronic infective mastitis, duct ectasia, hematoma, and breast abscess. Malignant causes include DCIS, Paget disease of the breast, and neurosarcoma.

It is useful to test the discharge for occult blood. In a study of patients undergoing microdochectomy for a discharge that could be localized to a single duct, all 16 patients with an occult cancer had a positive test for occult blood. Of the 268 benign lesions, 69 produced a discharge that was negative for blood and 199 produced a discharge that was positive.

The discharge was not tested in eight cases (Chaudary et al, 1982). In an earlier study, all 27 cases that tested negative for blood had a benign cause (Atkins and Wolff, 1964).

Then skipping a paragraph of questions, we come to "it is not prudent to withhold a simple test (a biopsy) on the basis of a few small studies. *Breast surgeon Lanfranchi would biopsy patients with a discharge having ANY* [I capitalized, numbered, and italicized this] *of the following PATHOLOGICAL features*: [1] *spontaneous* (noticed on bra or nightgown); [2] *involves one breast* [unilateral] *or one duct*; [3] *serous or bloody* in character; or [4] *associated with a mass*. If ALL these criteria are fulfilled, the risk of cancer is about 10%. Features indicating a benign cause are occurrence a) only when the doctor squeezes [provided his name is not erased from the registry – oh, that's me again] (some discharge can be expressed in 60% of women); b) bilateral; c) involves multiple ducts; d) colored; or, e) not associated with a mass (A. Lanfranchi, personal communication, 2009)."

So in Arizona, they are recommending nipple expression too! Expert 1, now doesn't this sound like the very information that you failed to bring forward from the Monica Morrow article that you chose to only partially quote from in the *American Family Practitioner Journal*? Do you happen to know who this Lanfranchi guy is? Most of our readers will just notice that his name isn't yours. He is quoted in the world literature. Yours is not! You might come across his name, if ever you did a real literature search. Committee members, is the state of Arizona camouflaging their ill intent by shrouding it with such a technique?

So, Mr. Registrar and his expert, *do you do CME to keep up with medicine*? Do you judge others based on what you learn? Mme L'Expert, everyone now knows that you claimed to have done *an extensive literature search* on this subject. You are obviously really bad at literature searches, extensive or otherwise. I'm not sure anyone is going to be able to believe you if you preface your remarks with that assurance.

Finally, now, here is a quote from Mark Swartz 2010, *Textbook of Physical Diagnosis*, sixth edition. Mark is from *New York*. From his chapter 16, "The Breast," page 469 [bottom of page]:

EXAMINE THE NIPPLE

> Examination of the nipple concludes the examination of the breast. Inspect for nipple retraction, fissures, and scaling. To examine for discharge, place each hand on either side of the nipple and gently compress [squeeze] the nipple, noting the character of <u>any</u> discharge. This technique is demonstrated in Figure 16-20. Ask the woman whether she would prefer to perform *this part of the examination* herself. [Most will decline; I have asked. But the offer is very politically correct by today's standards.]

Now, some parting words to the college, especially the registrar and his key expert witness. I have brought you quotes from some of the *best textbooks of physical examination in the world*. I hope you have had your eyes opened if you operated in ignorance. If you did not operate in ignorance, then how can you live with yourselves? These texts were chosen, not because if you dig deep enough you can find anything, but because they are all on the shelves of the University of Alberta Medical Bookstore where expert 1 attended.

Now, guess which textbook of physical examination is recommended by the *New England Journal of Medicine*. [I'll bet *even you two* have heard of that journal!] Well, of course, it has been the Swartz textbook for the last ten years or more. I suggest it's time to go back to school – with the registrar, Mme L'Expert.

Back to *A Knight's Tale*. Standing over Adhemar [whom I so see as our dear registrar].
Wat: You have been weighed.
Roland: You have been measured.
Kate: And you have absolutely . . .
Chaucer: *Been found wanting!*

William: Welcome to a New World. God save you, *if it is right that he should do so.*

Oh, and by the way, as I said, I picked up all of these texts at the bookstore at the University of Alberta. But the attendant says that for some reason, students are still only buying the Bates text. Sometimes what is done by a traditional medical school is just too traditional. Would it not be wise to ask a student to master two approaches, at least. There is a big world out there, and *"we're not the only deer in the forest"* (from *Bambi*).

There are some traditions in medical schools that should probably be abandoned. So what about the traditions around the complaints process and disciplinary hearings at colleges? Do those "traditions" compromise the fairness of the process? Could there be things that everyone just does during the process that actually render it unfair from within (see my chapter 6)? Although I have been treated destructively and have been actually required to pay very dearly for this assault and pain, I would like to spend my last chapter constructively.

CHAPTER 10

WHAT CAN YOU LEARN FROM MY EXPERIENCE ABOUT SURVIVING YOUR HOLOCAUST?

THE COLLEGE OF Some Physicians and Two Surgeons of Alberta printed in their newsletter, *The Messenger*, for June 2008 that council had found me guilty of demonstrating a lack of skill, judgment, or unbecoming conduct for

1. manipulating the nipples of the breasts of one patient, on March 9, 2000, and one patient on March 21, 2001 in an effort to express secretions "when there was no medical reason for doing that . . ." [And now every reader knows that there is a common, recommended, and purposeful reason.]

2. examining the back of one patient April 3, 2001, one patient September 1, 2001, and one patient December 30, 2001 in such a manner that my (left) hand contacted the bare breast of that patient [after having assessed that specific physical exam technique as of March 5, 2000, and providing me their formal

written impression that it was not out of line with normal practice];

3. doing a pelvic exam on April 10, 2001, and December 30, 2001 on two patients: one as a follow-up exam which a <u>seasoned surgeon</u> would not have done in one instance [Does everyone now believe that that her view is considered the standard for all <u>family doctors</u> in Alberta?]; and, in the other, in a situation in which an Osteopath would not have done it, explaining that he would have referred the exam to someone else [In the second instance there was also to have been NO prior explanation. Pretty sketchy grounds for that one too, as we've shown.];

4. performing manual therapy without obtaining ANY consent [but definitely giving the college-required running commentary]; and

5. undoing the brassiere of a patient to expose her back for a back exam [which the only course in Canada on physician boundaries says is not just appropriate but mandatory in abiding the spirit of appropriate doctor-patient boundaries].

It was upon these "proven (?)" allegations, and these alone, that they figured I should be erased from the register. That was the plan wasn't it, gang?

Now, these readers have more than just the take of the registrar, Counsel for the College, and incorrect expert witnesses on these five specific "shortcomings." Do you think that they might be noticing more than just MY shortcomings – *actually, noticing YOUR shortcomings*? Don't you worry that some of the lesser players in your production are going to feel somewhat compromised? Some may want an explanation from you. They may feel used or exploited. Might those two young women who have had such troubled lives, now feel that the office of registrar has contributed to their misery by misinformation? So what will you do now that they and these readers are aware – expecting ethical guidance? They pretty well know that

I can't sue any of you. I even have to be cautious that *my description, of your defamation of my character, cannot somehow be construed as my defamation of your character.* Now *that's ironic, isn't it*! In the end it is probably TRUE that each of us defames our own character to whatever degree that it is defamed! Have you besmirched your own characters and the office that you hold? So what will you now do to avoid further self-defamation? What are the *ETHICAL THINGS that you should now do?*

From my side, shall I just call you all bad names? I suspect no one would blame me. But my final message here has to be founded in my ethics, not yours. When I was in practice, I never did hang up my degrees, diplomas, and licenses because if I didn't have the answers, then all that wallpaper wouldn't help my patients, either. What do your walls look like? I love the Toronto Western Hospital motto: "There is always an answer! We will find it!" What will you do next? It's something over which I have no control. I will try to be at peace, remembering, "God *grant me the serenity to accept the things I cannot change.*"

The next lines in this prayer are, "The courage to change the things I can, and the wisdom to know the difference." I must go on. I must live and become employed at something. I am going back to school, but until then I am working at a bakery and pruning trees. It is very hard work, but it is honest. I now know through personal experience what my previously oft-used in medicolegal letters phrase "work hardening" means. We do what we need to do. We harden. Life is not fair. We don't have the luxury of waiting for life to become fair. It just never is going to be fair. That was never guaranteed: get used to it! If we just stand and shake our fists at heaven, we eventually are going to be tired and hungry, as are those who depend upon us. Stop crying, but you may weep because unfairness is pretty sad. Make friends if you don't have any. Join a faith group if you are not already a part of one. Get a job if you haven't one. Keep close to your family, and enjoy the time you have with them. They are of worth! Really notice them. They are good. Work to make your most intimate relationship keep going, or consider creating one. A pet will rarely betray you, and puppies are really nice. Especially one named Kevin! Oh, she's a Morkie, and she's a girl dog. I speak to you as one who has felt the stinging winds of oppression in his face. If you are in such a storm now, know that others HAVE been there. Create for yourselves a network of support. You are really worth having around.

Now, on a more personal note: *Mr. Registrar,* everyone who reads this will know that even if you did not personally do everything that was wrongly done in this "hearing," the buck stops with you. You end up being responsible. You wanted to be the registrar; you accepted the responsibility. All of this happened *on your watch.* [*Remember I served in the military.*]

Though as a brother I can forgive you, I cannot excuse you. You have personally hurt me and my family and my patients. Those patients are the ones who wrote and asked you to let me continue to attend them in spite of your "findings." Remember? Yet I still want to encourage you, even implore you, to do better. The profession that you have been given some power over is a NOBLE one. Don't taint it further.

Make sure that you personally KNOW the teachings of physical exam that are legitimate BEFORE you judge them. Otherwise you will break our first oath: <u>TO DO NO HARM</u>! To inform a complaining patient that something that she complains of was, in your view, of an assaultive and inappropriate nature directly harms her, if you are wrong.

Further, while you do control the employment of so many within the college itself and within the province, you are also being watched. Whereas, you may have been bullied yourself at some point in your own life, don't use this position to get even. It doesn't become you.

You may wish to talk *with me* at some time, man-to-man, instead of ensuring that someone else does it *for you.*

And you, my former lawyer, actually did have expert 1 acknowledging that she would like to know the *date of the book* that showed that nipple expression was appropriate. I don't know if you knew of her shaky honesty at the time because you certainly didn't pursue it. But you did finally get her to ask the question that showed that she had been aware that publications of "older date" [and, as we have learned here, of newer date too] did make that recommendation. You just didn't follow it up. That left me dangling on the razor edge of the "goodwill" of the college. And they had none toward me.

<u>To my ex-patients who tried to stick with me as my ship was torpedoed and sunk,</u> thank you for your loyalty! Thank you for letting me be a part of your lives. You have honored me! I enjoyed my service to you. My medical techniques were not self-serving.

"Think of me, think of me fondly – as I will think of you! Remember me once in a while . . ." (from *The Phantom of the Opera* by Andrew Lloyd Webber).

There are those of you who came to me over the years and asked that I not do certain parts of exams on you. I believe I was faithful in allowing you that freedom, although I did not necessarily agree with your choices. Find someone else who will tolerate your wishes yet still attend you. You are of worth.

Know this, that I did my best for you – every time! I love you guys! I would not have missed our relationship for the world. Serving you was an honor. Before she died, Dianne asked me, "Bry, if you knew then what challenges there would be, would you still have chosen medicine over law?" To which I answered, "Absolutely!" And she said, "I'm glad, me too!" See, I told you she was supportive. I saw her tombstone in place for the first time today, May 25, 2010.

Who really can predict what will be the outcome now? The committee felt that I hadn't demonstrated *adequate remorse* for what they believed were my actions. If I had done those actions, I certainly would be remorseful. I didn't do them, as you have learned. Yet I was not perfect. I know I am human. Even if I became a doctor, I was not right all the time. But the numerous life mistakes I have made are still mine alone to know. *What I am remorseful about* is that the con-woman and her friend were so willing to change, modify, and embellish their stories. And I am remorseful that the college seemed to countenance those fictitious stories. I am, also, remorseful that two very uncertain young women became *pawns of whom further advantage was taken* by the hearing process. I suspect that they are no better off now than they were when I first started seeing them – not because of me, but because of the process they became caught in. What will become of them? What will become of me? *What will I do* now?

I know that I will *trudge along*. While we were still together, Dianne asked that if she die, I remarry. Those conversations were painful, then, and painful now as I recall them. Sometimes she would point out a certain person that she felt *she* would be compatible with – for me to marry after her passing. I always thought that I would just have a heart attack on my way into the hospital for a delivery. And I assumed that it would be I who would go first.

Early in the history of the faith that Dianne and I embraced, there had been 3 percent of the brethren who practiced plural marriage. I can easily say that to be married to and grow with *one* spouse is challenge enough. Yet I believe it is for our best in this life. Biggest challenge – best for us! Definitely hard work, but worth it! And in ways perhaps beyond my comprehension, Dianne sacrificed for me. While in the course of these proceedings – so fraught with err – I tried to go to work and continue to see patients. My ankles were swelling and aching at the end of the day often. And then, they began to *not stop aching* by the time the next day began. For weeks this continued. When I came home one day from work, Dianne asked me how my ankles had felt THAT day. I said they had improved for the first time in weeks, and she informed me that she had prayed and asked if she would be allowed to carry that burden for me. She told me that her own ankles had started aching and swelling that day, but that *she was happy* that her prayers had been heard. Oh my goodness! I am still left in awe of her!

I haven't dated for many years. I tried to dutifully go out with the ladies that Dianne had pointed out as "okay by her." I'm really bad at dating now. Maybe I always was. When one of my wife's chosen "ladies" called and cancelled a date due to a migraine, I tried to be supportive and call to follow up that she was okay. Because she was not available. I just hung up and called back later. That's how I remember doing things when I was a "little dater," and also I have this doctor thing about headaches. Our technologies are so advanced that she could scan and see that I had attempted to call six times. When she finally did speak to me, she gave me the impression that she thought I was *stalking her*! She seemed to articulate a fear of me. That hurt – yes, *somehow I can still be hurt*. In all fairness, she has never been married and enjoyed the caring and concern that is associated with that honorable union. No, I wasn't stalking. *Why would I want to find someone who did not want to find me?* Perhaps I will never find someone: one last impact of the <u>rule of thirds</u>!

No, I won't be doing any stalking. I will mostly be *trudging* as you've read from my quote from Chaucer earlier. Perhaps I will publish small books about things I used to talk with my patients about. Like the "rules of coexistent living" – how families or roommates can live best together, or like "cycles of relationship." And I will be trying to find work, possibly in the field of research, because I *am* a researcher and student of medicine. Well, that is what I do, but not entirely who I am. My name is Bryant Litchfield, and I am a person – just like you. I refuse to spend my days shaking my fist at heaven for my poor lot. I am not mad at God for taking my wife. I am grateful to Him for having let me have her at my side for thirty-two years. She brought me through this trial. She had my back every step of the way. I am so thankful to Him for letting her be my wife. She is busy doing things somewhere else. She still encourages me. She still exists. I still exist. Perhaps, somewhere in the future of existence, I will have earned the right to be with her again. Perhaps I will have remarried. If so, it must be to someone I know would be compatible with Dianne. Perhaps, if God choose, Dianne – "*I shall but love thee better, after death*!" (Quoted from Elizabeth Barrett-Browning's *How Do I Love Thee?*.)

Now I have to tell you that the writing of this history has been a part of my healing. My writing is not likely to change much, the unethical proceedings that occurred. But I hope that they enable to live more at peace. Perhaps you should consider writing your own stories or, if it would help, send me an account of your trial. I am not here to condemn, and I probably can't change your situation, but I can listen. I am good at listening!

Lastly, there will be those of you who will still get "taken into some alley by a bully." Accusations, just like bullying, tend to isolate you from your peers, your friends, and your safety. Examine yourself when this happens. If you are at peace that the accusations or singling out are wrong, then JUST HOLD ON! If they are right, then change yourself. You can change things in this generation! Bad stuff doesn't have to be "passed on" and on.

Start to trudge – exercise will help you. *Continue or start to eat as if you deserved to be treated properly.* Don't join with the bully – who is a part of everything that is wrong! Please, accept some encouragement from me, if no one else is there for you. Dianne still encourages me. *The light is there.* When they are in plain sight, bullies usually go quiet. They like to be aggressive, but passively (unseen), because they are not very brave.

****

INDEX

www.ingramcontent.com/pod-product-compliance
Lightning Source LLC
Chambersburg PA
CBHW031836170526
45157CB00001B/319